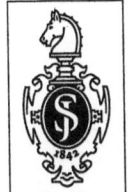

S. Andò   C. Brancati   (Eds.)

Endocrine Disorders in Thalassemia

Physiopathological and Therapeutical Aspects

With the Collaboration of
M. Maggiolini, G. De Luca and M. Bria

With 39 Figures, Some in Color
and 42 Tables

Springer-Verlag
Berlin Heidelberg New York
London Paris Tokyo
Hong Kong Barcelona .
Budapest

Prof. Dr. Sebastiano Andò
Head of Endocrine Physiopathology Unit
University of Calabria
Department of Cellular Biology
87030 Arcavacata di Rende (CS)
Italy

Prof. Dr. Carlo Brancati
Head of Experimental Medicine and Biotechnology Institute
C.N.R. Cosenza
Via Fratelli Cervi No. 1
87100 Cosenza
Italy

ISBN-13:978-88-470-2185-3   e-ISBN-13:978-88-470-2183-9
DOI: 10.1007/978-88-470-2183-9

Library of Congress Cataloging-in-Publication Data
Endocrine disorders in thalassemia: physiological and therapeutic aspects/S. Andò, C. Brancati (eds.): with the collabora-
tion of M. Maggioloni, G. De Luca, and M. Bria. p. cm. Includes index.
ISBN-13:978-88-470-2185-3
1. Thalassemia – Endocrine aspects. 2. Thalassemia – Complications. 3. Endocrine glands – Diseases. I. Andò, S.
(Sebastiano), 1948 – II. Brancati, C. (Carlo), 1924 – RC641.7.T5E53 1994/616.1'52 – dc20

Typesetting: E. Kieser, D-86356 Neusäß
SPIN 10123088   65/3130 5 4 3 2 1 0 – Printed on acid-free-paper

Preface

Since in the past 20 years new therapeutic trends (hypertransfusion regimen and iron chelation therapy) have greatly improved the life expectancy of thalassemics, endocrine abnormalities may develop and worsen the quality of life of these patients.

This volume represents the updated proceedings of the "International Mediterranean Conference on Endocrine Disorders in Thalassemia," held May 7–9, 1992, in Cosenza and organized by the University of Calabria and by the CNR. The Conference was the first dealing extensively with the most frequent endocrine abnormalities of thalassemic patients; it focused on such topics as growth and growth hormone, thyroid diseases, puberty, hypogonadism, bone metabolism and diabetes.

The practical objective of the Conference was to give an opportunity to people working in this field and coming from countries with different socioeconomic conditions to meet, to share their experiences, and to establish guidelines for the management of endocrine disorders in thalassemia major. This is in agreement with a fundamental requirement of medical ethics: that any progress we make in research into a certain illness should be passed on to all those suffering from it, guaranteeing them the same therapeutic benefits and the same quality of life. Thus it becomes increasingly important to make a new therapeutic approach equally available to all thalassemic patients, and this really does require national and international cooperation in hemoglobinophathy programs.

It is our hope that the Conference will lead to the setting up of a multicenter study, the results of which may be presented at subsequent scientific meetings promoted by some of the other countries involved. The aim should be to achieve a better understanding of the factors that probably determine the incidence of endocrine diseases in thalassemic patients of different countries, as well to assess the efficacy of the therapeutic approach and any fallout in terms of quality care.

We wish to thank all the participants and all the scientists who came to Cosenza for their active contribution, making the "International Mediterranean Conference on Endocrine Disorders in Thalassemia" a really successful congress. Our special thanks go to Dr. Vincenzo De Sanctis for his excellent scientific coordination of the conference. Finally, we express our gratitude for the prestigious organizational support we enjoyed from the Community of Mediterranean Universities.

S. ANDÒ
C. BRANCATI

Contents

Communications

List of Contributors

AKAR, N., Pediatric Hematology and Endocrinology Departments of Ankara
University, Büklüm sokak 20/8, 06660 Kavaklidere, Ankara, Turkey

ALEXANDRIDES, T. K., Department of Medicine, Medical School of Patras,
University Hospital of Patras, Rion-Patras 26500, Greece

AL-FAWAZ, I., Medical Biochemistry Department (30), College of Medicine
and King Khalid Hospital, P. O. Box 2925, Riyadh 11461, Saudi Arabia

AL-QADREH, A., Thalassemia Unit, Microbiology Laboratory and Institute
of Child Health, Aghia Sophia Children's Hospital, Athens, Greece

ANASTASI, S., Thalassemia Unit, Department of Pediatrics, Garibaldi Hospital,
Catania, Italy

ANDÒ, S., Health Center and Department of Cellular Biology, University
of Calabria, Italy

ANDRADE, A., Growth Unit, General Hospital of Vigo, P. O. Box 1691,
36201 Vigo, Spain

ANGELUCCI, E., Divisione di Ematologia e Centro Trapianto di Midollo Osseo di
Muraglia, Ospedale di Pesaro, Italy

APONTE, S., XXIX Pediatrics Division, Cardarelli Hospital, Via Netti, 36,
80131 Naples, Italy

AQUILA, S., Health Center, University of Calabria, Italy

ARCASOY, A., Pediatric Hematology and Endocrinology Departments of Ankara
University, Büklüm sokak 20/8, 06660 Kavaklidere, Ankara, Turkey

ARMONI, A., Medical School of Patras, University Hospital of Patras, Rion-Patras
26500, Greece

AZIZLERLI, H., Social Security Göztepe Hospital, Medical School Istanbul, Turkey

BAGNI, B., Servizio di Medicina Nucleare, USL 31, Arcispedale S. Anna,
Corso Giovecca 203, 44100 Ferrara, Italy

BAGNI I., Servizio di Medicina Nucleare, USL 31, Arcispedale S. Anna,
Corso Giovecca 203, 44100 Ferrara, Italy

BALDUCCI, R., Laboratorio Centrale Ospedale di Pesaro, Italy

BARONCIANI, D., Divisione di Ematologia e Centro Trapianto di Midollo Osseo di
Muraglia, Ospedale di Pesaro, Italy

BARTSOCAS, C. S., First Department of Pediatrics, P. & A. Kyriakou Children's
Hospital and Biochemistry Laboratory, University of Athens, 6 Faiakon St.,
175 63 – P. Faliro, Greece

BISCONTE M. G., CNR-Hematology Center, Cosenza, Italy

BONACCORSI, G., Servizio di Medicina Nucleare, USL 31, Arcispedale S. Anna, Corso Giovecca 203, 44100 Ferrara, Italy

BONESCHI, A. L., Clinica Ostetrico-Gynecologica, Ospedale S. Gerardo di Monza, via Solferino 16, 20052 Monza, Italy

Bouloukos, A., First Department of Pediatrics, P. & A. Kyriakou Children's Hospital and Biochemistry Laboratory, University of Athens, 6 Faiakon St., 175 63 – P. Faliro, Greece

BRANCATI, C., Experimental Medicine and Biotechnology Institute C. N. R., 87100 Cosenza, Italy

BRAUNER, R., Unité 30, Hôpital Necker-Enfants-Malades, Paris, France

BRIA, M., CNR – Hematology Center, Cosenza, Italy

CANTONE, M., Thalassemia Unit, Department of Pediatrics, Garibaldi Hospital, Catania, Italy

CARACCIOLO, M., CNR – Hematology Center, Cosenza, Italy

CARUSO, V., Thalassemia Unit, Department of Pediatrics, Garibaldi Hospital, Catania, Italy˙

CARUSO-NICOLETTI, M., Clinica Pediatrica II, Università di Catania, V. le A. Doria, 95125 Catania, Italy

CAVALLINI, A. R., Servizio di Medicina Nucleare, USL 31, Arcispedale S. Anna, Corso Giovecca 203, 44100 Ferrara, Italy

CAVALLO, L., Dipartimento di Biomedicina dell'Età Evolutiva, Università di Bari, Policlinico, Piazza G. Cesare, 11, 70124 Bari, Italy

CHATTERJEE, R., Reproductive Medicine Unit, Department of Obstetrics and Gynaecology, University College and Middlesex School of Medicine, 86–96 Chenies Mews, London WC1E 6HX, U. K.

CHATZILIAMI, A., Thalassemia Unit, Microbiology Laboratory and Institute of Child Health, Aghia Sophia Children's Hospital, Athens, Greece

CONSARINO, C., Servizio di Microcitemia ed Emopatie Infantili, Ospedale A Pugliese, Catanzaro, Italy

CORCIONI, E., Hospital of Rogliano, Cosenza, Italy

D'ANGELO, P., Prevention and Care Center for Thalassemia, Pediatric Department, Villa Sofia Hospital, Palermo, Italy

De Luca, G., Health Center, University of Calabria, Italy

De Mattia, D., Dipartimento di Biomedicina dell'Età Evolutiva, Università di Bari, Policlinico, Piazza G. Cesare, 11, 70124 Bari, Italy

DE MONTALEMBERT, M., Service d'Hématologie, Hôpital Necker-Enfants-Malades, Paris, France

DE SANCTIS, V., Department of Pediatrics, Arcispedale, S. Anna, Corso Giovecca 203, 44100 Ferrara, Italy

DI GREGORIO, F., Centro di Microcitemia, Università di Catania, viale A. Doria, 95125 Catania, Italy

DI MAIO, S., Department of Pediatrics, Università Federico II, Naples, Italy

EL-HAZMI, M., Medical Biochemistry Department (30), College of Medicine and King Khalid Hospital, P. O. Box 2925, Riyadh 11461, Saudi Arabia

ERER, B., Divisione di Ematologia e Centro Trapianto di Midollo Osseo di Muraglia, Ospedale di Pesaro, Italy

FADINI, R., Clinica Ostetrico-Gynecologica, Ospedale S. Gerardo di Monza,
   via Solferino 16, 20052 Monza, Italy
FILOSA, A., XXIX Pediatrics Division, Cardarelli Hospital, Via Netti, 36,
   80131 Naples, Italy
FONTOURA, M., Unité 30, Hôpital Necker-Enfants-Malades, Paris, France
FRAGODIMITRI, C., Thalassemia Unit, Microbiology Laboratory and Institute
   of Child Health, Aghia Sophia Children's Hospital, Athens, Greece
GALATI, M. C., Servizio di Microcitemia ed Emopatie Infantili,
   Ospedale A Pugliese, Catanzaro, Italy
GALIMBERTI, M., Divisione di Ematologia e Centro Trapianto di Midollo Osseo
   di Muraglia, Ospedale di Pesaro, Italy
GAMBERINI, M. R., Department of Pediatrics, Arcispedale S. Anna, Corso Giovecca
   203, 44100 Ferrara, Italy
GARCÍA-MAYOR, R. V., Growth Unit, General Hospital of Vigo, P. O. Box 1691,
   36201 Vigo, Spain
GAZIEV, J., Divisione di Ematologia e Centro Trapianto di Midollo Osseo
   di Muraglia, Ospedale di Pesaro, Italy
GERTNER, J., New York Hospital-Cornell Medical Center, Division of Pediatric
   Hematology/Oncology, 525 East 68th Street, New York, NY 10021, USA
GIANNAKI, M., Thalassemia Unit, Microbiology Laboratory and Institute of Child
   Health, Aghia Sophia Children's Hospital, Athens, Greece
GIARDINA PATRICIA J., New York Hospital-Cornell Medical Center,
   Division of Pediatric Hematology/Oncology, 525 East 68th Street, New York,
   NY 10021, USA
GIARDINI, C., Divisione di Ematologia e Centro Trapianto di Midollo Osseo
   di Muraglia, Ospedale di Pesaro, Italy
GIOBBE, T., Dipartimento di Biomedicina dell'età Evolutiva, Università di Bari,
   Policlinico, Piazza G. Cesare, 11, 70124 Bari, Italy
GIORDANO G., DISEM, Cattedra di Endocrinologia, Università di Genova,
   viale Benedetto XV, 6, 16100 Genova, Italy
GIORNO, A., Health Center, University of Calabria, Italy
GIROT, R., Service d'Hématologiem Hôpital Necker-Enfants-Malades, Paris, France
GIUSTI, M., DISEM, Cattedra di Endocrinologia, Università di Genova,
   viale Benedetto XV, 6, 16100 Genova, Italy
GIUZIO, E., Clinica Ortopedica Facoltà di Medicina, Università Federico II,
   Naples, Italy
GÖKÇEN, Ö., Social Security Göztepe Hospital, Medical School Istanbul, Turkey
GONI, MARIE-HELENE, Department of Endocrinology, Hippokration Hospital,
   108 Vas. Sophias Ave., 115–27 Athens, Greece
GRIMALDI, S., Servizio di Microcitemia, Crotone, Italy
GUIDO, R., DISEM, Cattedra di Endocrinologia, Università di Genova,
   viale Benedetto XV, 6, 16100 Genova, Italy
HANSLIP, J. I., Department of Haematology, Whittington Hospital, Highgate Hill,
   London N19 5NF, England
HAZANI, A., Rambam Medical Center, Haifa, Israel

HILGARTNER, MARGARET W., New York Hospital-Cornell Medical Center, Division of Pediatric Hematology/Oncology, 525 East 68th Street, New York, NY 10021, USA

HOCHBERG, Z., Faculty of Medicine, Technion, P.O. Box 9649, Haifa 31096, Israel

Italian Working Group of Endocrine Complications in Non-Endocrine Diseases

JOUSEF, J., Thalassemia Unit, Microbiology Laboratory and Institute of Child Health, Aghia Sophia Children's Hospital, Athens, Greece

KAFOUROU, A., First Department of Pediatrics, P. & A. Kyriakou Children's Hospital and Biochemistry Laboratory, University of Athens, 6 Faiakon St., 175 63 – P. Faliro, Greece

KANADIKIRIK, F., Social Security Göztepe Hospital, Medical School Istanbul, Turkey

KARABATSOS, F., Thalassemia Unit, Microbiology Laboratory and Institute of Child Health, Aghia Sophia Children's Hospital, Athens, Greece

KARAGIORGA-LAGANA, M., Thalassemia Unit, Microbiology Laboratory and Institute of Child Health, Aghia Sophia Children's Hospital, Athens, Greece

KATSANTONI, A., Thalassemia Unit, Microbiology Laboratory and Institute of Child Health, Aghia Sophia Children's Hospital, Athens, Greece

KATZ, M., Department of Obstetrics and Gynaecology, University College and Middlesex School of Medicine, 86–96 Chenies Mews, London WC1E 6HX, U.K.

LANZI, E., Patologia Medica, Ospedale S. Gerardo di Monza, via Solferino 16, 20052 Monza, Italy

LANZINO, M., Department of Cellular Biology, University of Calabria, Italy

LESSER, M., New York Hospital-Cornell Medical Center, Division of Pediatric Hematology/Oncology, 525 East 68th Street, New York, NY 10021, USA

LEUZZI, R., Dipartimento di Biomedicina dell'Età Evolutiva, Università di Bari, Policlinico, Piazza G. Cesare, 11, 70124 Bari, Italy

LIUZZI, S., Dipartimento di Biomedicina dell'Età Evolutiva, Università di Bari, Policlinico, Piazza G. Cesare, 11, 70124 Bari, Italy

LO IACONO, F., Prevention and Care Center for Thalassemia, Pediatric Department, Villa Sofia Hospital, Palermo, Italy

LO PINTO, C., Prevention and Care Center for Thalassemia, Pediatric Department, Villa Sofia Hospital, Palermo, Italy

LO PRESTI, D., Clinica Pediatrica II, Università di Catania, via le A. Doria, 95125 Catania, Italy

LUCARELLI, G., Divisione di Ematologia e Centro Trapianto di Midollo Osseo di Muraglia, Ospedale di Pesaro, Italy

LUNA, R., Endocrine Division, General Hospital of Vigo, P.O. Box 1691, 36201 Vigo, Spain

MAGGIOLINI, M., Health Center, University of Calabria, Italy

MAGNANO, C., Thalassemia Unit, Department of Pediatrics, Garibaldi Hospital, Catania, Italy

MAGRO, S., Servizio di Microcitemia ed Emopatie Infantili, Ospedale A Pugliese, Catanzaro, Italy

MAKRI, M., Medical School of Patras, University Hospital of Patras, Rion-Patras
26500, Greece

MALIZIA, R., Prevention and Care Center for Thalassemia, Pediatric Department,
Villa Sofia Hospital, Palermo, Italy

MALYALI, D., Social Security Göztepe Hospital, Medical School Instanbul, Turkey

MANCUSO, M., Clinica Pediatrica II, Università di Catania, via le A. Doria,
95125 Catania, Italy

MANCUSO, R., Servizio di Microcitemia ed Emopatie Infantili,
Ospedale A Pugliese, Catanzaro, Italy

MARKUSSIS, V., Department of Endocrinology, Hippokration Hospital,
108 Vas. Sophias Ave., 115–27 Athens, Greece

MICALIZZI, C., Hematology and Oncology Department, Gaslini Institute, Genova,
Italy

MIGNINI-RENZINI, M., Clinica Ostetrico, Gynecologica, Ospedale S. Gerardo
di Monza, via Solferino 16, 20052 Monza, Italy

MISASI, M., Clinica Ortopedica Facoltà di Medicina, Università Federico II,
Naples, Italy

MONGUZZI, W., Clinica Pediatrica, Ospedale S. Gerardo di Monza,
via Solferino 16, 20052 Monza, Italy

MORGIONE, S., Servizio di Microcitemia ed Emopatie Infantili,
Ospedale A Pugliese, Catanzaro, Italy

MORI, P. G., Hematology and Oncology Department, Gaslini Institute, Genova, Italy

NEW MARIA, New York Hospital-Cornell Medical Center, Division of Pediatric
Hematology/Oncology, 525 East 68th Street, New York, NY 10021, USA

NOUNOPOULOS, H., First Department of Pediatrics, P. & A. Kyriakou Children's
Hospital and Biochemistry Laboratory, University of Athens, 6 Faiakon St.,
17563 – P. Faliro, Greece

ÖKAL, G., Pediatric Hematology and Endocrinology Departments of Ankara
University, Büklüm sokak 20/8, 06660 Kavaklidere, Ankara, Turkey

PANEBIANCO, V., Clinica Pediatrica II, Università di Catania, via le A. Doria,
95125 Catania, Italy

PARAMO, C., Endocrine Division, General Hospital of Vigo, P. O. Box 1691,
36201 Vigo, Spain

PÉREZ MENDEZ, L. F., Endocrine Division, General Hospital of Vigo,
P. O. Box 1691, 36201 Vigo, Spain

PERFUMO, F., Nephrology and Dialysis Department, Gaslini Institute, Genova, Italy

PÉRIGNON, F., Unité 30, Hôpital Necker-Enfants-Malades, Paris, France

PETROU, G., Medical School of Patras, University Hospital of Patras, Rion-Patras
26500, Greece

PEZZI, V., Health Center, University of Calabria, Italy

PINAMONTI, A., Department of Pediatrics, Arcispedale S. Anna,
Corso Giovecca 203, 44100 Ferrara, Italy

PINTOR, C., Department of Pediatric Endicrinology, University of Cagliari, Italy

PITROLO, L., Prevention and Care Center for Thalassemia, Pediatric Department,
Villa Sofia Hospital, Palermo, Italy

POLCHI, P., Divisione di Ematologia e Centro Trapianto di Midollo Osseo di Muraglia, Ospedale di Pesaro, Italy

PORTER, J. B., Department of Haematology, University College and Middlesex Hospital Medical School, 86–96 Chenies Mews, London WC1E 6HX, U. K.

POSTEL-VINAY, M. C., INSERM, Unité 344, Hôpital Necker-Enfants Malades, Paris, France

PUZZONIA, P., Servizio di Microcitemia ed Emopatie Infantili, Ospedale A Pugliese, Catanzaro, Italy

RAIOLA, G., Divisione di Pediatria, Ospedale A Pugliese, Catanzaro, Italy

RAPPAPORT, R., Unité 30, Hôpital Necker-Enfants-Malades, Paris, France

RIVOLTA, M. R., Clinica Medica, Ospedale S. Gerardo di Monza, via Solferino 16, 20052 Monza, Italy

RODRIGUEZ, AMANDA, New York Hospital-Cornell Medical Center, Division of Pediatric Hematology/Oncology, 525 East 68th Street, New York, NY 10021, USA

ROMEO, F., Servizio di Anatomia Patologica, Ospedale Civile, Cosenza, Italy

RUDOLF, MARY C. J., Rambam Medical Center, Haifa, Israel

SABATO, V., Dipartimento di Biomedicina dell'Età Evolutiva, Università di Bari, Policlinico, Piazza G. Cesare, 11, 70124 Bari, Italy

SANTILLI, E., Servizio di Microcitemia ed Emopatie Infantili, Ospedale A Pugliese, Catanzaro, Italy

SAVIANO, A., XXIX Pediatrics Division, Cardarelli Hospital, Via Netti, 36, 80131 Naples, Italy

SCHETTINI, F., Dipartimento di Biomedicina dell'Età Evolutiva, Università di Bari, Policlinico, Piazza G. Cesare, 11, 70124 Bari, Italy

SCHNEIDER, R., New York Hospital-Cornell Medical Center, Division of Pediatric Hematology/Oncology, 525 East 68th Street, New York, NY 10021, USA

SHEHADEH, N., Rambam Medical Center, Haifa, Israel

SIMMONS, B., New York Hospital-Cornell Medical Center, Division of Pediatric Hematology/Oncology, 525 East 68th Street, New York, NY 10021, USA

SISCI, D., CNR – Health Center, University of Calabria, Italy

SKORDIS, N., Department of Paediatrics, Makarios Hospital, Nicosia, Cyprus

SONAKUL, D., Department of Pathology, Siriraj Hospital, Bangkok 10700, Thailand

SPADARO, G., Clinica Pediatrica II, Università di Catania, V. le A. Doria, 95125 Catania, Italy

SPANOS, E., First Department of Pediatrics, P. & A. Kyriakou Children's Hospital and Biochemistry Laboratory, University of Athens, 6 Faiakon St., 175 63 – P. Faliro, Greece

SPILIOTIS, B. E., Medical School of Patras, University Hospital of Patras, Rion-Patras 26500, Greece

SPROCATI, M., Department of Pediatrics, Arcispedale S. Anna, Corso Giovecca 203, 44100 Ferrara, Italy

STAMOGIANNOU, L., First Department of Pediatrics, P. & A. Kyriakou Children's Hospital and Biochemistry Laboratory, University of Athens, 6 Faiakon St., 175 63 – P. Faliro, Greece

TAPAKI, G., Thalassemia Unit, Microbiology Laboratory and Institute of Child Health, Aghia Sophia Children's Hospital, Athens, Greece

THEOCHARI, MARIA, First Department of Pediatrics, P. & A. Kyriakou Children's Hospital and Biochemistry Laboratory, University of Athens, 6 Faiakon St., 175 63 – P. Faliro, Greece

TINNIRELLO, G., Clinica Pediatrica II, Università di Catania, V. le A. Doria, 95125 Catania, Italy

TOLIS, G., Department of Endocrinology, Hippokration Hospital, 108 Vas. Sophias Ave., 115–27 Athens, Greece

TRENTADUE, F., Dipartimento di Biomedicina dell'Età Evolutiva, Università di Bari, Policlinico, Piazza G. Cesare, 11, 70124 Bari, Italy

TUTAR, H. E., Pediatric Hematology and Endocrinology Departments of Ankara University, Büklüm sokak 20/8, 06660 Kavaklidere, Ankara, Turkey

UGHI, M., Department of Pediatrics, Arcispedale S. Anna, Corso Giovecca 203, 44100 Ferrara, Italy

VALENTI, S., DISEM, Cattedra di Endocrinologia, Università di Genova, viale Benedetto XV, 6, 16100 Genova, Italy

VERO, A., Servizio di Radioimmunologia, Ospedale A Pugliese, Catanzaro, Italy

VULLO, C., Department of of Pediatrics, Arcispedale S. Anna, Corso Giovecca 203, 44100 Ferrara, Italy

WARSY, A., College of Science, King Saud University, Riyadh, Saudi Arabia

WONKE, BARBARA, Department of Haematology, Whittington Hospital, Highgate Hill, London N19 5NF, U.K.

Plenary Lectures

Spontaneous Growth Hormone (GH) Secretion and Results of Therapy with GH in Thalassemic Patients

Z. Hochberg, M. C. J. Rudolf, N. Shehadeh, and A. Hazani

Life expectancy for patients with thalassemia major (TM) has greatly improved, and their hopes are now directed towards attainment of better quality of life. The growth retardation of many of these patient becomes a major concern for the patients, their families, and the medical care-giver.

Growth retardation of children with TM is multifactorial; it can be the consequence of chronic hypoxia, liver disease, anorexia, hypothyroidism, hypogonadism, and dysfunction of the growth hormone (GH)-IGF-I axis. Analysis of the growth curves of TM patients discloses onset of deviation from the normal growth curve during late childhood, towards the end of the first decade of life. This may imply a role for impairment of the GH-IGF-I axis. Indeed, GH response to GHRH has been shown to be impaired, and serum IGF-I is low, while GH response to provocative stimuli is normal. GH-binding protein, as a measure of the GH receptor, is low, but not to an extent that may affect growth.

The present report therefore concentrates on the role of GH in the growth retardation of TM patients, their response to provocative GH stimulation, the 24-h spontaneous secretion of GH, and the effect of rhGH treatment.

GH Secretion

The subjects of this study were seven patients with TM, four female and three male, aged 6–16 years and prepubertal. They were on a hypertransfusion regimen to maintain their hemoglobin levels above 9 gm/dl, but none had received desferrioxamine therapy. Their growth rates were at or below -2 SD for their respective age. The control group was comprised of two sex- and age-matched individuals for each patient.

All seven TM patients had normal GH response to pharmacological stimulation by consequent administration of arginine (0.5 g/kg) and insulin (0.1 U/kg). Their peak GH was 9.6–23 µg/l, compared with control peak GH of 16 ± 3 µg/l.

The GH profile was carried out for 16–24 h in continuous fractions of 30 min. GH peak analysis was performed visually, by examining a plot of plasma GH against time, and by the PULSAR program. TM patients had fewer pulses during the collection period, with 1–5 pulses, compared with 6.5 ± 2 for the controls. The mean pulse amplitude was 6.3–10 µg/l in TM patients and 13 ± 3.2 µg/l in controls. The integrated concentration of GH was 1.9–3.2 µg/l in TM and 5.8 ± 1.3 in controls.

S. Andò et al. (Eds.)
Endocrine Disorders in Thalassemia
© Springer-Verlag Berlin Heidelberg 1995

Thus, TM patients have normal GH response to pharmacological stimulation, but marked subnormal spontaneous secretion of GH. This pattern of response corresponds with the definition of neurosecretory dysfunction of GH secretion [1].

A more critical view of the data infers that five of the patients had delayed puberty, which might have contributed to the low spontaneous GH secretion. Indeed, hypogonadism is a common endocrinopathy in TM patients, and future research needs to account for that variable by appropriate controls, and by GH testing after priming with sex steroids.

rhGH Therapy

Results of the first phase of the study led to the thrapeutic trial of GH therapy in TM patients. Indeed, previous reports from our group and from others indicated a useful growth response to GH therapy in patients with low integrated concentrations of GH, and the response was negatively correlated with GH levels.

Five TM patients with slow growth and low spontaneous GH secretion were then treated with rhGH for 12 months. They were 11.3–17.4 years of age, three female and two male, with bone age of 7–15 years, height SDS of −2.8 to −5.2, and Tanner pubertal stage of 1–2. Three had hypothyroidism and were on L–T_4 replacement, two had hypoparathyroidism and were on vitamin D therapy and normocalcemic. They received rhGH in a dose of 0.07–0.09 IU/kg daily s.c. for 6 months. Growth velocity increased from 3.4 ± 1 to 4.8 ± 0.8 cm/year. As this response was judged to be insufficient, the GH dose was increased to 0.14–0.16 IU/kg daily. During the next 6 months the children grew at a rate of 5.6 ± 2 cm/year.

Whereas the increase in growth rate was statistically significant, the growth response to hGH therapy was judged to be very poor when compared with that of children with GH deficiency, normal short stature, or Turner's syndrome. Similar results were obtained by other investigators [2], which corresponds with the poor IGF-I response to short-term GH in such patients [3].

Conclusions

Results of the first phase of this report imply neurosecretory dysfunction of GH secretion in patients with TM, as defined by their normal response to pharmacological stimulation tests for GH secretion, but subnormal spontaneous GH secretion. This led us to the second phase, in which we administered GH to such patients and observed a statistically significant response, that was, however, disappointing in terms of attainment of absolute growth rate improvement.

A critical review of our own results indicate that five of the seven phase-1 patients and four of the five phase-2 patients had delayed puberty. A similar review of the results of Scacchi et al. [2] indicates that their patients also had delayed puberty. This condition, which is very common in TM [4], is also associated with impairment of GH secretion. Delayed puberty is a matter of social concern for adolescents, and they deserve appropriate therapy with sex steroids at a suitable age, to allow them to mature with their peers. Our present approach is to treat children with TM and delayed puberty with low-dose sex steroids, beginning at 12 years of age for girls and at 13 years of age for boys. With such treatment we have observed acceleration of growth that is comparable to that observed with GH therapy (unpublished).

We therefore presently feel that the endocrinopathy that is responsible for the growth retardation of most TM patients is delayed puberty, or hypogonadotropic hypogonadism, which provokes a secondary decrease in GH secretion. The preferred treatment of such patients is therefore low-dose sex steroids, rather than GH. This mode of therapy allows the TM child with delayed puberty and growth retardation to mature with his peers and to undergo a growth spurt at a normal age.

References

1. Shehadeh N, Hazani A, Rudolf MCJ, Peleg I, Benderly A, Hochberg (1990) Neurosecretory dysfunction of growth hormone secretion in thalassemia major. Acta Paediatr Scand 79: 790–795
2. Scacchi M, Danesi L, De Martin M, Dubini A, Forni L, Masala A, Gallisai D, Burrai C, Terzoli S, Boffa C, Marzano C, Cavagnini F (1991) Treatment with biosynthetic growth hormone of short thalassemic patients with impaired growth hormone secretion. Clin Endocrinol (Oxf.) 35: 335–339
3. Werther GA, Matthews RN, Burger HG, Herington AC (1981) Lack of response of non-suppressible insulin-like activity to short-term administration of human growth hormone in thalassemia major. J Clin Endocrinol Metab 53: 806–809
4. Johnston FE, Hertzog KP, Malina RM (1966) Longitudinal growth in thalassemia major. Am J Dis Child 122: 396–399

Plasma Growth Hormone-Binding Protein and Liver Receptor in Thalassemic Patients

M. C. Postel-Vinay, M. Fontoura, M. de Montalembert, F. Pérignon, R. Brauner, R. Rappaport, and R. Girot

Children with thalassemia major often present with growth failure, the mechanism of which is not clear. They are not GH deficient but their plasma insulin-like growth factor I (IGF_I) activity is markedly reduced [1–5]. Therefore, the cause of the growth defect is likely to be at the GH receptor or post-receptor level: in either case it would lead to impairment of GH-induced generation of IGF_I.

To test the hypothesis of a GH receptor binding defect, the plasma GH-binding protein (GHBP) was evaluated in thalassemic patients. The amino acid sequences of GHBP and of the extracellular domain of the GH receptor are identical [6]; thus GHBP is a soluble, short form of the membrane GH receptor. Many questions regarding biosynthesis, function, and regulation of GHBP have yet to be elucidated. However, GHBP represents the only possible approach to the GH receptor in man, in vivo, and its level probably reflects the liver GH receptor concentration.

Subjects

Twenty-one patients (14 girls, 7 boys) with thalassemia major were studied. They were separated into two groups. *Group 1* consisted of 14 patients aged 6–14 years, all prepubertal. Among them, nine had received a low transfusion regimen, without chelation therapy, and five patients had a high transfusion regimen and received chelation therapy. *Group 2* consisted of seven patients aged 14–20 years, all pubertal. They all had been treated with a high transfusion regimen and correct chelation therapy. All patients had growth failure, as presented in Table 1.

Measurement of GHBP

Binding of 125 I-hGH to plasma GHBP was determined as previously described by Tar et al. [7]. Briefly, plasma (100 µl) was incubated for 20 h at 4 °C with 100 µl potassium phosphate 0.1 M, pH 7.0, BSA 0.1 %, containing 125 I-h-GH (2×10^5 c.p.m.). After filtration through a 0.45-mm Millipore minifilter, the entire incubation mixture was injected onto a HPLC Protein Pak 300 sw column(0.75 x 30 cm). Elution was performed isocratically using a degassed buffer (Na_2SO_4 0.1 M, potassium phosphate 0.1 M, pH 7.0) pumped at a rate of 0.5 ml/min. Radioactivity was recorded on-line using a Berthold LB 504 gamma detector connected to a computer.

S. Andò et al. (Eds.)
Endocrine Disorders in Thalassemia
© Springer-Verlag Berlin Heidelberg 1995

Table 1. GHBP determinations in thalassemic patients

	Sex	Age	GHBP (% of radioactivity)[a]	Height (SD)[b]
Group 1	M	6	17.5	− 1.5
	M	7	14.3	− 2.5
	M	7	23.5	− 2
	F	8	28.4	− 3.5
	M	8	19.8	− 1.5
	F	9	46.4	− 2
	F	10	21.2	− 3
	F	11	28.2	− 2.5
	F	11	31.9	− 2
	M	11	25.5	− 1
	F	12	26.4	− 2
	F	12	22.3	− 1
	F	13	29.6	− 1
	F	14	19.5	− 2
		mean ± SEM	23.3 ± 2.1	− 1.96 ± 0.20
Group 2	F	14	31.2	− 2
	F	16	21.3	− 1.7
	M	16	35.8	mean
	M	17	25.8	− 2.5
	M	17	30.5	− 2.2
	F	18	21.1	− 0.5
	F	20	19.6	− 2
		mean ± SEM	26.4 ± 2.3	− 1.56 ± 0,.35

[a] Normal GHBP value for age is 24.8 ± 1.7 % of radioactivity for group 1 and 27.2 ± 1.7 for group 2.
[b] Height is presented as SD from normal height.

The binding of hGH is expressed as the radioactivity in the individual peak divided by the total radioactivity in peaks, I, II, and III. To evaluate nonspecific binding to peak II-BP, 5 µg of GH was added to the plasma incubation.

Hormone Radioimmunoassays

hGH was measured by a double antibody method; Ist IRP hGH (WHO 66/217) was used for the standard. IGF_I was measured by RIA on acid-ethanol-extracted plasma.

Results and Discussion

The results of the GHBP determination are shown in Table 1. In the two groups, the mean GHBP value was comparable to the value found in age-matched normal subjects.

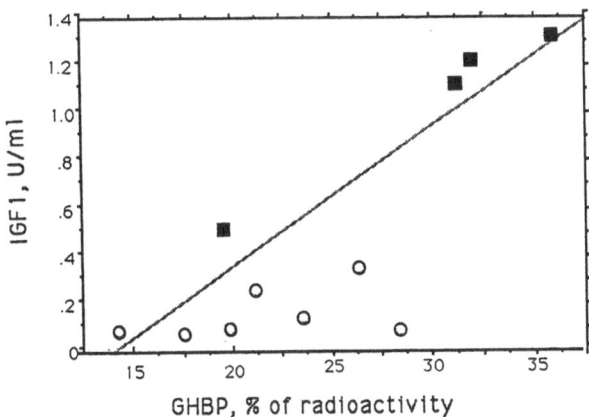

Fig. 1. Correlation between GHBP and IGF_I plasma levels in thalassemic patients. *Open circles*, values for patients with low transfusion regimen; *dark squares*, values for patients who received high transfusion regimen ($r = 0.806$, $p < 0.01$)

IGF_I plasma levels were determined in 11 patients. Figure 1 shows the positive correlation between IGF_I and GHBP plasma levels. IGF_I levels were low, except in three patients who received a high transfusion regimen. Decreased IGF_I plasma concentrations have previously been reported in thalassemic children, based on measuring either bioassayable [3, 4] or radioimmunoassayable IGF_I [5].

In man, the GHBP is probably produced through proteolysis of the membrane receptor [6, 8]. GHBP, like the cell membrane GH receptor, is regulated by multiple factors, among which GH itself has an important role [9]. The mechanism of the GHBP regulation will not be fully understood until more is known about the enzyme which is involved in the proteolysis of the membrane receptor.

Many examples from animal studies suggest that the GH binding activity measured in plasma reflects the level of hepatic GH receptors. Our studies of GH receptors in thalassemia also support this fact: thalassemic proteins have a normal plasma GHBP level, and we had previously shown that the GH binding level to their liver membrane was normal [10]. We took advantage of a liver biospy done for histological evaluation at the time of splenectomy. Part of the biopsy was used to prepare a membrane fraction by differential centrifugation, and the binding of 125 I-hGH to the liver membrane fraction was assessed. A large variation was found in the level of GH binding. However, the range of GH binding was comparable among thalassemic patients to that among normal transplant donors whom we were also able to study. No relationship was found between the level of GH binding to liver membranes and the severity of growth failure in the 17 patients whom we studied [10].

In conclusion, patients with thalassemia major have normal plasma GHBP activity and normal levels of GH binding to liver membrane fractions. Thus, the cause of the growth failure presented by the patients is not at the GH receptor level. Possible defects in post-receptor events cannot be eliminated. This study also demonstrates that the chance of better growth with a normal GHBP and IGF_I plasma level is greater in patients receiving a good transfusion regimen and iron chelation therapy.

References

1. Lassman MN, O'Brien RT, Pearson HA et al. (1974) Endocrine evaluation in thalassemia major. Ann NY Acad Sci 232: 226–231
2. Canale VC, Steinberg P, New MJ, Erlandson M (1974) Endocrine function in thalassemia major. Ann NY Acad Sci 232: 333–345
3. Saenger P, Schwartz E, Markenson AL et al. (1980) Depressed serum somatomedin activity in β-thalassemia. J Pediatr 96: 214–218
4. Herington AC, Werther GA, Matthews RN, Burger HGH (1981) Studies on the possible mechanism for deficiency of nonsuppressible insulin-like activity in thalassemia major. J Clin Endocrinol Metab 52: 393–398
5. Leger J, Girot R, Crosnier H, Postel-Vinay MC, Rappaport R (1989) Normal growth hormone (GH) response to GH-releasing hormone in children with thalassemia major before puberty: a possible age-related effect. J Clin Endocrinol Metab 69: 453–456
6. Leung DW, Spencer SA, Cachianes G et al. (1987) Growth hormone receptor and serum binding protein: purification, cloning and expression. Nature 330: 537–543
7. Tar A, Hocquette JF, Souberbielle JC, Clot JP, Brauner R, Postel-Vinay MC (1990) Evaluation of the growth hormone-binding proteins in human plasma using high-pressure liquid chromatography gel filtration. J Clin Endocrinol Metab 71: 1202–1207
8. Kelly PA, Djiane J, Postel-Vinay MC, Edery M (1991) The prolactin/growth hormone receptor family. Endocr Rev 12: 235–251
9. Postel-Vinay MC, Hocquette JF et al. (1991) Human plasma growth hormone-binding proteins are regulated by growth hormone and testosterone. J Clin Endocrinol Metab 73: 197–202
10. Postel-Vinay MC, Girot R, Léger J et al. (1989) No evidence for a detect in growth hormone binding to liver membranes in thalassemia major. J Clin Endocrinol Metab 68: 94–98

Short-term Follow-up Study of Thyroid Function in Polytransfused Thalassemic Patients

S. Andò, M. Maggiolini, G. De Luca, M. Bria, D. Sisci, M. Lanzino,
S. Aquila, V. Pezzi, A. Giorno, M. Caracciolo, M. G. Bisconte,
E. Corcioni, and C. Brancati

Among the endocrine abnormalities involving thalassemic patients, the incidence of thyroid disorders shows a large variability [1–8]. We attempted to investigate the evolutive trend of thyroid function with elapsing of time and its relationship with chelation therapy. We have carried out a follow-up study of thyroid function in 45 polytransfused thalassemic patients, investigated in 1988 and again in 1992.

Material and Methods

Patients

Forty-five polytransfused thalassemic patients (8–35 years old; 23 female and 21 male) and 25 healthy subjects (14 female and 11 male) in the same age range used as controls were studied. The thyroid function was evaluated in 1988 and 4 years later by determining total and free thyroid hormones (TT4, TT3, FT3, FT4), reverse T3 (rT3), thyroglobulin (Tg), thyroxine-binding globulin (TBG), thyroglobulin (AAT) and microsomal (AAM) antibodies, and thyrotropin (TSH) in basal conditions and 30, 60, 90, 120 min after a standard dose of TRH (200 µg i.v.). In the latter period (1992), aside from the hormonal-metabolic determinations, thyroid morphological evaluation with ultrasound was also performed on some thalassemic patients randomly selected ($n = 13$).

Hematological-Metabolic Parameters

Before each investigation the following parameters were checked in each patient, here expressed as mean value of almost three determinations: hemoglobin pretransfusional levels, ferritin serum levels, blood transfused units/year, desferrioxamine administered by subcutaneous infusions with portable microinfusers (mg/kg/day), the ratio iron chelated/transfusional iron introduced as chelation index, the number of the infusions in a year as chelation compliance, daily urinary iron excretion, and AST and ALT transaminase activities [9]. Hemoglobin levels were measured by an automatic counter (Coulter Counter S-Plus Jr, Hialea, Florida, USA). Ferritin serum levels were assayed by the immunoenzymatic method (Enzymum test, Boehringer Mannheim, Germany). Urinary iron excretion was evaluated by the colorimetric

S. Andò et al. (Eds.)
Endocrine Disorders in Thalassemia
© Springer-Verlag Berlin Heidelberg 1995

method (Enzycolor-Sibar, Poli Diagnostici, Milano, Italy). AST and ALT transaminase activities were measured by the spectrophotometric method (Refloton system, Boehringer Mannheim, Germany.

Hormonal-Metabolic Parameters

Total and free thyroid hormones (TT4, TT3, FT3, FT4), reverse T3 (rT3), thyroglobulin (Tg), thyroxine-binding globulin (TBG), thyroglobulin (AAT) and microsomal (AAM) antibodies, thyrotropin (TSH) in basal conditions and 30, 60, 90, 120 min after a standard dose of TRH (200 µg i.v.) were measured. The TSH release to TRH administration was evaluated as maximal level achieved (mxv) as well as integrated area of response (ϵ). In the presence of thyroid hormone levels mantained in the normal range, a maximal value of TSH upon TRH more than 1 SD over control mean was considered an index of subclinical hypothyroidism [10, 11]. Serum TSH and Tg were measured by IRMA-sensitive commercial kits (Byk-Sangect, Germany). Serum TT4, TT3, rT3, and TBG were assayed by RIA commercial kits (Baxter, Cambridge, USA; Byke-Sangect, Germany; Radim, Rome Italy. Serum FT3 and FT4 were measured by RIA commercial kits with preliminary chromatographic separation (Tecnogenetics, Milan, Italy). AAT and AAM were assayed with an RIA-coated tube (Biodata, Italy and Sorin Biomedica, Italy). Values > 100 U/ml were considered positive results for AAT and values > 10 U/ml were considered positive results for AAM. The intraassay and interassay C.V. were $< 10\%$ in all previous determinations.

Ultrasound Evaluation

Ultrasound evaluation of thyroid volume was carried out on 13 (5 female and 8 male) randomly selected patients in 1992 and in 15 healthy controls (7 female and 8 male), according to the criteria of Chanoine et al. [12]. The volume of each lobe was calculated separately using the formula of an ovoid (depth x length x width x $\pi/6$). The total thyroid volume represents the value of both lobes.

Statistical Analysis

Statistical analyses were carried out with Students's t-Test and Pearson's correlation.

Results

No significant differences of hormonal metabolic values were found in either thalassemics or controls grouped according to sex and age; thus the individual data of each hormonal-metabolic parameter investigated have been pooled and expressed as a mean value. In 1988 hormonal mean levels were not significantly different with respect to controls (Table 1). Individual values revealed that of the 45 thalassemic subjects studied, one male patient (2.2%) exhibited clear hormonal features of overt hypothyroidism, i.e., TSH basal value extremely high (55 m IU/l), low T3 (0.6 ng/ml), and T4 (27 ng/ml), and one female patient (2.2%) dispayed an increase of TSH release to TRH consistent with subclinical hypothyroidism, as reported in Material and Methods.

No significant changes in hematological-metabolic parameters were revealed in the time elapsing between the two tests, while significant changes in thyroid function were observed (Table 2). Indeed, of 44 patients tested again in 1992, four (2 female and 2 male) developed overt hypothyroidism (9%) and 14 (8 female and 6 male) displayed a subclinical hypothyroidism (31.8%) with reduced FT3 levels $(3.3 \pm 0.7$ pg/ml vs C 5.3 ± 0.3, $p < 0.01$), resulting in a lower FT3/FT4 molar ratio $(0.38 \pm 0.1$ vs C 0.8 ± 0.16, $p < 0.001$). It is interesting to note that in the patients developing subclinical hypothyroidism the FT3/FT4 molar ratio in 1992 was significantly reduced with respect to the earlier investigation $(88:0.7 \pm 0.27$ vs $92:0.38 \pm 0.1)$.

Thus, at the end of the present investigation five subjects (11.1%) were affected by overt hypothyroidism and 15 (33.3%) by subclinical hypothyroidism. It is worthy of note that the group of patients developing subclinical hypothyroidism during the follow-up study displayed at both investigations a significant increase of ALT trans-aminase activity with respect to the remaining patients $(88:62.8 \pm 13.7$ vs 30.5 ± 6.16 IU/l, $p < 0.01$; $92:45 \pm 9.2$ vs 26 ± 3.6 IU/l, $p = 0.02$) and in 1992 an increase of ferritin levels $(3282 \pm 585$ vs 2096 ± 266 ng/ml, $p = 0.03$) which appeared positively related to AST and ALT concentrations $(r = 0.7$; $p < 0.01$).

In 1988 as well as in 1992, thyroglobulin and microsomal antibodies were below the positivity limit in all patients. Similarly, no thalassemic subject presented goiter at either investigation.

The thyroid volume randomly evaluated by ultrasound in eight euthyroid thalasse-mic sujects (5 female and 3 male), in three patients with subclinical hypothyroidism (2 female and 1 male) and in two patients with overt hypothyroidism (1 female and 1 male) was greatly reduced with respect to 15 healthy controls (7 female and 8 male) (Th: 5.5 ± 4.2 ml vs C: 15.2 ± 2.3, $p < 0.001$) and negatively related to TSH maximal value $(r = -0.66$; $p < 0.02$) as well as to its integrated area of response to TRH $(r = -0.68$; $p < 0.02$). It is noteworthy that patients displayng overt hypo-thyroidism and two of those developing subclinical hypothyroidism showed a thyr-oid volume clearly below the lower value of euthyroid thalassemic patients (Fig. 1).

The gland size bore no correlation with the ferritin levels of the same patients. For instance, it is interesting to observe that in one patient with greatly elevated ferritin levels (3240 ng/ml) the thyroid volume was maintained (10.8 ml).

Discussion

According to recent reports, thalassemic patients living in Mediterranean countries still have a low compliance with iron chelation therapy [4, 5]. Our data show that

Table 1. Hormonal – metabolic parameters (X ± SEM) evaluated in the same thalassemic patients in 1988 and 1992 and in 25 control subjects

	bv TSH (mIU/l)	mxv TSH	s TSH	T3 (ng/ml)	T4 (ng/ml)	FT3 (pg/ml)	FT4 (pg/ml)	rT3 (ng/dl)	TBG (µg/ml)	HTg (ng/ml)	AAT (U/ml)	AAM (U/ml)
C (n 25)	1.66 ± 0.4	13 ± 1.9	632.7 ± 30.1	1.9 ± 0.06	82.7 ± 5.2	5.3 ± 0.3	9.2 ± 0.3	19.7 ± 0.1	22.3 ± 0.1	18.2 ± 1.8	31 ± 1.8	3.9 ± 0.42
Th '88 (n 44)	2.4 ± 0.3	12.3 ± 1.1	688 ± 66**	1.4 ± 0.07	76 ± 4.8	4.6 ± 0.2	8.6 ± 0.4	18 ± 0.2	10. ± 0.2	20 ± 2.8	42 ± 2.5	5.9 ± 0.5
Th '92 (n 40)	2.1 ± 0.2	19.1 ± 1.3	1234 ± 107**	1.5 ± 0.08	72.4 ± 2.5	4.1 ± 0.6	8.3 ± 0.5	16.9 ± 0.3	19.2 ± 0.1	34.2 ± 4.8	48.1 ± 2.7	5.2 ± 0.3

bv TSH, basal value TSH; *mxv TSH* maximal value achieved by TSH upon TRH; ε *TSH*ˣ integrated area of TSH response to TRH; *C*, controls; *Th*, thalassemic patients.
*p < 0.01; **p < 0.001

Table 2. Hematological – metabolic parameters (X ± SEM) evaluated in 44 thalassemic patients in 1988 and 1992

	Hb (gr/dl)	UT (year)	Fe (ng/ml)	DS (mg/kg/day)	I.Ex. (mg/Day)	Ch. In.	Co. In.	AST (UI/l)	ALT (UI/l)
Th '88 (n 45)	10.3 ± 0.1	24.4 ± 0.8	2651 ± 261	28.9 ± 1.3	1.3 ± 0.9	1.4 ± 0.2	0.65 ± 0.02	22.1 ± 2.3	30.1 ± 3.7
Th '92 (n 45)	10.1 ± 0.1	22.2 ± 0.7	2501 ± 282	30.7 ± 1.1	15.4 ± 1.6	1.24 ± 0.1	0.68 ± 0.02	16.7 ± 1.6	32.2 ± 4.2

*Hb*ˣ, Hemoglobin pretransfusional levels; *UT*ˣ, blood transfused units; *Fe*ˣ, serum ferritin levels; *DS*ˣ, desferrioxamine administered; *I.Ex.*ˣ, daily urinary iron excretion; *Ch.In.*ˣ, Chelation Index; *Co. In.*ˣ, compliance index; *Th*, thalassemic patients.

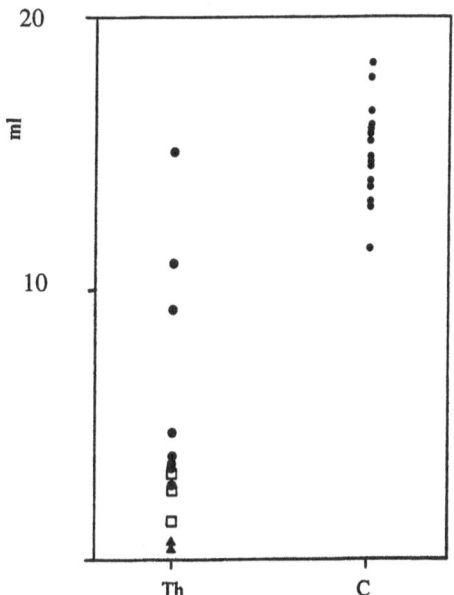

over time thalassemic patients may develop thyroid disorders with varying degrees of severity. Indeed, of the 44 patients tested again in 1992, four developed overt hypothyroidism and 14 displayed an augmented TSH response to TRH administration consistent with subclinical hypothyroidism. Thus the incidence of overt (11.1%) and subclinical (33.3%) hypothyroidism had greatly increased by the end of our investigation.

The thyroid ultrasound evaluation revealed reduced glandular volumes which appeared unrelated to ferritin circulating levels. In order to explain the latter findings we have to consider that with the passage of time, the iron store in the thyroid tissue can induce glandular damage by the synthesis of collagen fibers, leading to autonomous progressive fibrotic change in the endocrine parenchyma [13].

A serum ferritin concentration up to 4000 ng/ml seems to be directly correlated to the hepatic iron deposit: 1 mg/l of serum ferritin is equivalent to 1 mg/g dry weight of liver iron, although such an equation should not be applied to a single value, above all not in the presence of liver disease [14, 15]. Indeed, chelation therapy is not simultaneously involved in the changes of serum ferritin since its concentration usually decreases 12–24 mounths after the start of treatment with desferrioxamine [16].

Thus, ferritin circulating levels in a large sample of thalassemic patients represent a general index for evaluating iron overload, whereas the individual serum ferritin concentration is unable to provide an estimate of iron accumulation in the various organs because iron distribution is certainly not homogeneous.

An impairment of liver function in subjects developing subclinical hypothyroidism was supported by the greater enhancement of transaminase levels with respect to euthyroid patients. In the same patients in 1992, both transaminase values appeared positively related to ferritin levels, very likely of an indication of how hepatic hemosiderosis progressively affects liver function. It is interesting to note that the patients with unchanged rT3 levels displayed an FT3 and FT3/FT4 molar ratio that was markedly decreased with respect to that observed 4 years earlier. On the basis of the above-reported observations, we suggest a possible hepatic influence per se on thyroid function and/or on the hormonal peripheral metabolism, as previously shown in patients with other liver diseases [17]; for instance, the extrathyroid conversion rate of T4 to T3 has been found lowered in liver dysfunction [18]. Thus, we may speculate that in the subgroup of patients developing subclinical hypothyroidism the impaired liver function could reduce the activity of hepatic iodothyronine 5' monodeiodinase, leading to the lowering of FT3 levels.

The absence of thyroglobulin and microsomal antibodies at the two investigations in all subjects revealed that autoimmune mechanisms do not seem to contribute to the impairment of thyroid function, as previously reported [7]. The reduced thyroid function was not associated in any patient with a glandular enlargement evaluated by palpation, very likely because the local iron store had led to volumetric regression.

We may thus conclude that:

1. An impairment of thyroid function with different degrees of severity, without goiter, frequently occurs in thalassemic patients of both sexes.
2. An impaired liver function leads to a probable extraglandular component of thyroid disease.
3. The absence of thyroid antibodies seems to exclude autoimmune mechanisms in such an endocrine complication.
4. A moderate compliance with chelation therapy does not seem to protect patients from thyroid dysfunction.
5. A periodical thyroid evaluation is a useful tool for setting up a therapeutic treatment in order to prevent overt hypothyroidism.

References

1. Landau H, Spitz IM, Cividalli G, Rachmilewitz EA (1978) Gonadotrophin, thyrotrophin, and prolactin reserve in β-thalassaemia. Clin Endocrinol(oxf), 9: 163–173
2. Madeddu G, Dore A, Marongiu A, Langer Costanzi M (1978) Growth retardation, skeletal maturation and thyroid function in children with homozygous β-thalassemia. Clin Endocrinol(oxf), 8: 359–365
3. Costin G, Kogut MD, Hyman C, Ortega JA (1979) Endocrine abnormalities in thalassemia major. AmJ Dis Child 133:497–502
4. De Sanctis V, Pintor C, Aliquo S, Anastasi S, Borgna-Pignatti C, Brancati C et al. (1990) Preliminary data on prevalence of endocrine complications in patients with β-thalassemia major: an Italian multicenter study. In: (Pintor C, Corda R, De Sanctis V) (eds) Porto Cervo, Sardinia Workshop on Endocrine Problems in Thalassemia, Oct 11
5. De Sanctis V, Pintor C, Andò S, Aliquò MC, Anastasi S, Brancati C et al. (1992) Prevalence of endocrine complications in patients with β-thalassemia major: an Italian multicenter study. International Mediterranean Conference on Endocrine Disorder in Thalassemia, May 7–9, Cosenza
6. Livadas D, Sofroniadou K, Souvatzoglou A, Boukis M, Siafaka L, Koutras D (1984) Pituitary and thyroid insufficiency in thalassemic haemosiderosis. Clin Endocrinol(oxf), 20: 435–443

7. Phenekos C, Karamerou A, Pipis P, Constantoulakis M, Lasaridis J, Detsi S, Politou K (1984) Thyroid function in patients with homozygous β-thalassemia. Clin Endocrinol(oxf) 20: 445–450

8. Bisbocci D. Sperone D, Camaschella C, Bertero T, Livorno P, Degani G, D'Alberto M (1987) Hyperresponsiveness of plasma TSH to TRH and thyroid antibodies in postpubertal clinically euthyroid patients with thalassemia major. Ital 3: 47–52

9. Modell B, Berdoukas V (1984) Iron overload – desferrioxamine. In: The clinical approach to thalassemia. Grune and Stratton, Orlando, pp 198–240

10. Bartalena L, Bogazzi F, Pinchera A (1991) Thyroid function tests and diagnostic protocols for investigation of thyroid dysfunction. Ann Ist Super Sanita 27 (3): 531–540

11. Bogner U, Arntz HR, Peters H, Schleusener H (1993) Subclinical hypothyroidism and hyperlipoproteinaemia: indiscriminate L-thyroxine treatment not justified. Acta Endocrinol (Copenh) 128: 202–206

12. Chanoine JP, Toppet V, Lagasse R, Spehl M, Delange F (1991) Determination of thyroid volume by ultrasound from the neonatal period to adolescence. Eur Pediatr 150: 395–399

13. Weintraub LR, Goral A, Grasso J, Franzblau C, Sullivan A, Sullivan S (1988) Collagen biosynthesis in iron overload. Ann NY Acad 526: 179–184

14. Worwood M, Cragg SJ, Jacobs A, McLaren C, Ricketts C, Economidou J (1980) Binding of serum ferritin to concanavalin A: patients with homozygous β-thalassemia and transfusional iron overload. Br Haematol 46: 409–416

15. Cazzola M, Borgna-Pignatti C, Då Stefano P, Bergamashi G, Bongo IG, Dezzá L, Avato F (1983) Internal distribution of excess iron and sources of serum ferritin in patients with thalassemia. Scand Haematol 30: 289–296

16. Cohen A, Martin M, Schwartz E (1981) Response to long-term desferrioxamine therapy in thalassemia. J Pediatr 99: 689–694

17. Long RG (1980) Endocrine aspects of liver disease. Br Med J 1: 225–228

18. Chopa IJ (1987) Alterations in thyroid physiology in liver disease. Serono Symp Publ 43: 157–164

Spermatogenesis in Patients with β-Thalassaemia major and intermedia

M. Katz, V. De Sanctis, C. Vullo, B. Wonke, M. Ughi, A. Pinamonti, M. Sprocati, M. R. Gamberini, and B. Bagni

Treatment of thalassaemia has improved to the exent that about 55 % of boys and girls with homozygous β-thalassaemia now enter puberty normally with the assurance of greater longevity and with the prospect of future marriage. For these reasons, many new problems are emerging to challenge doctors who care for patients with thalassaemia. The purpose of this study was to evaluate the fertility potential of thalassaemic men who have achieved full sexual maturation, either spontaneously or on treatment with gonadotrophins.

Materials and Methods

Semen analysis was performed in 47 patients with β-thalassaemia major and ten with thalassaemia intermedia who were being regularly or occasionally followed up in Ferrara and London. The age of patients with β-thalassaemia major varied between 15 and 33 years, that of patients with thalassaemia intermedia between 16 and 28 years.

Testicular volume, using Prader's orchidometer, ranged from 12 to 25 ml in most patients, but five patients with thalassaemia major and one with thalassaemia intermedia had testicular volumes between 10 and 12 ml. The diagnosis of homozygous β-thalassaemia was made on the basis of clinical and laboratory findings [1].

All patients with β-thalassaemia major received regular blood transfusions from the time of diagnosis, with the aim of mantaining their pretransfusion haemoglobin concentrations between 10 and 11 g/dl. The haemoglobin levels in patients with thalassaemia intermedia ranged from 7 to 8.5 g/dl and only a few received occasional blood transfusions.

To minimize tranfusional iron overload desferrioxamine mesylate (Desferal, Ciba-Geigy) was administered intramuscularly to patients with β-thalassaemia major up to 1979. After 1979, desferrioxamine was given by subcutaneus infusion for 10–12 h per day (20–50 mg/kg body wt.)

The serum ferritin levels in patients with β-thalassaemia major ranged from 205 to 7572 ng/ml, with a median of 1078 ng/ml. In patients with thalassaemia intermedia, serum ferritin levels ranged from 240 to 3400 ng/ml (Fig. 1).

Twenty-one patients with β-thalassaemia major (aged 16–21 years) who had hypogonadism or arrested puberty received gonadotrophin treatment to induce spermatogenesis. Human chorionic gonadotrophin (HCG, Profasi Serono), 2000 units,

S. Andò et al. (Eds.)
Endocrine Disorders in Thalassemia
© Springer-Verlag Berlin Heidelberg 1995

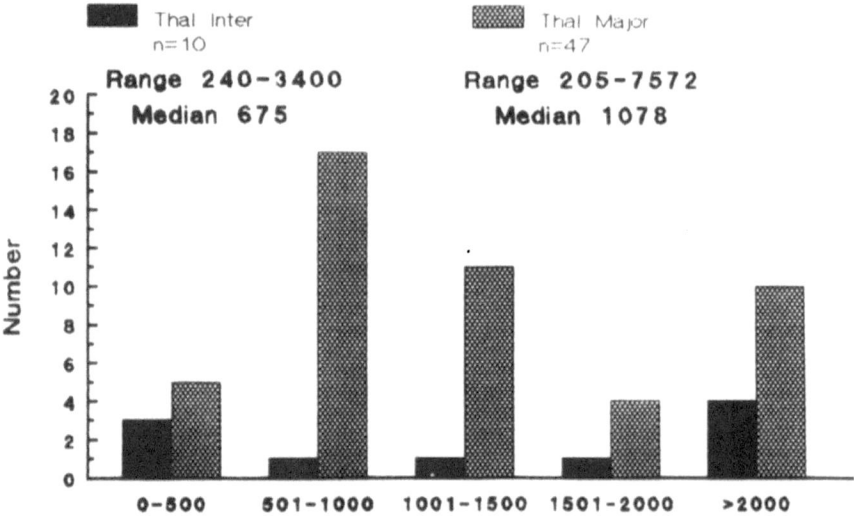

Fig. 1. Distribution of serum ferritin levels in patients with β-thalassaemia major and intermedia

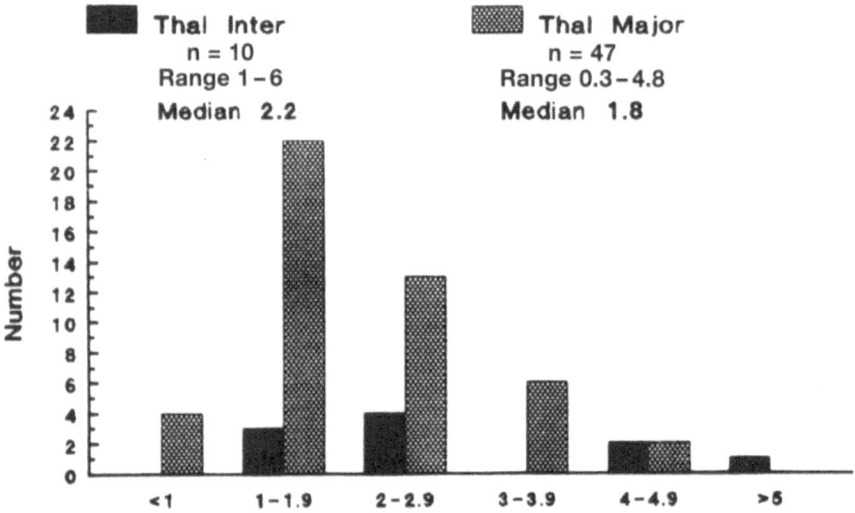

Fig. 2. Distribution of semen volume (ml) in patients with β-thalassaemia major and intermedia.

was administered intramuscularly twice weekly for 6 weeks to 14 months, until testosterone levels rose to the adult range (320–990 ng/dl). Then one ampule (75 IU) of human menopausal gonadotrophin (Pergonal, Serono) was added to the HCG regime three times a week.

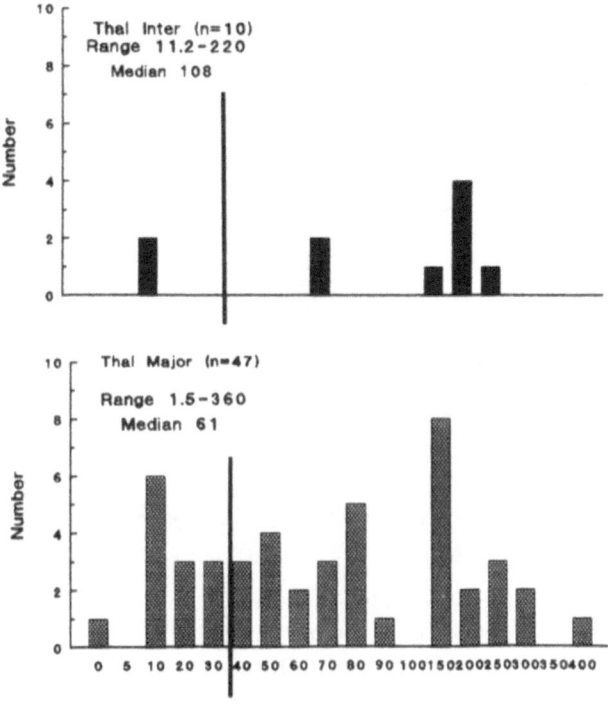

Fig. 3. Distribution of total sperm count (millions) in patients with β-thalassaemia major and intermedia

Semen parameters were assessed according to the recommendations of the World Health Organization [2]. Pituitary-gonadal function was evaluated in the basal state by immunoradiometric assay (IRMA) of luteinizing hormone (LH), follicle-stimulating hormone (FSH), and total and free testosterone (TT and FT). Serum ferritin levels were measured by radioimmunoassay (RIA; normal values 108 ± 69 ng/ml). Linear regression analysis was used to evelute correlations between variables.

Results

Thalassaemia major

The seminal volume in patients with thalassaemia major ranged from 0.3 to 4.8 ml (Fig. 2). Total sperm count varied from 1.5 million to 360,000,000, with a median of 61,000,000; 34% of patients (16/47) had a total sperm count below 42 million, the lower acceptable normal limit (Fig. 3). Similarly, taking 40% as the cut-off point for normal motility, 19% of the patients (9/47) had a low sperm motility.

Nineteen of 47 patients were followed up for 1–4 years. The sperm counts in nine were normal initially and remained normal; in two the counts, initially normal,

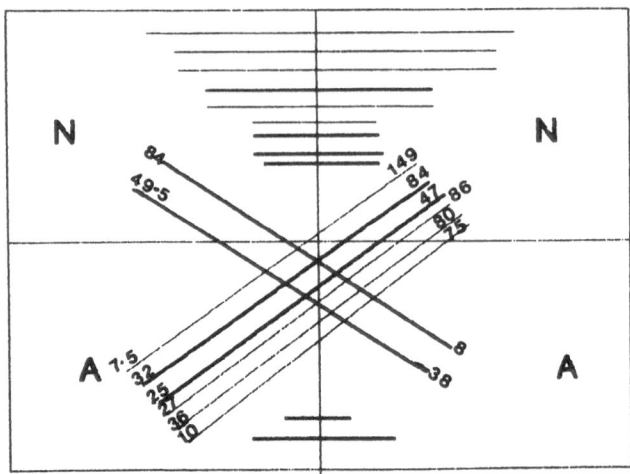

Fig. 4. Follow-up-study of total sperm counts in patients with β-thalassaemia major. Numbers refer to the sperm counts in patients with normal (*N*) and abnormal (*A*) sperm counts

diminished to abnormally low levels during the follow-up period, and in six low initial counts rose to the normal range during the follow-up (Fig. 4). Eleven of the 19 patients had normal percentage motility and three abnormal percentage motility both at their presentation and at follow-up. Another three had normal motility initially, which diminished into the abnormally low range at follow-up, and two had abnormal motility at presentation, which subsequently increased into the normal range (Fig. 5).

Where ferritin levels were 500 ng/dl or less, four of seven patients had low sperm counts and two had poor motility. Only one patient with a ferritin level below 500 ng/dl had a totally normal semen analysis.

No correlation was observed between total sperm count and ferritin concentration, FSH, LH, TT and FT, but there was a strong correlation between patient age and sperm count ($r = 0.45$, $p < 0.001$; Fig. 6).

Thalassaemia intermedia

With respect to thalassaemia intermedia, the seminal volume was normal in all patients (1–6 ml) (Fig. 2). The total sperm count and morphology were normal in seven of ten patients; count an motility were diminished in two patients and the count was normal, but the motility was reduced in one patient. During the follow-up of five patients for 1–4 years the sperm count and motility remained normal in one patient and abnormal in one and changed from abnormal to normal in one patient. Morphology was invariably normal in all patients.

No correlation was observed between sperm count and ferritin concentrations, FSH, and LH but there was a strong correlation with age, TT and FT ($r = 0.52$, 0.62, and 0.72; $p < 0.003$, < 0.05, and < 0.6, respectively).

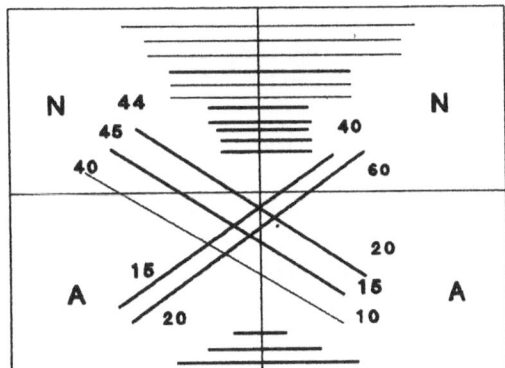

Fig. 5. Follow-up-study of sperm motility in patients with β-thalassaemia major. Numbers refer to per centage motility in patients with normal (*N*) and abnormal (*A*) sperm motilities

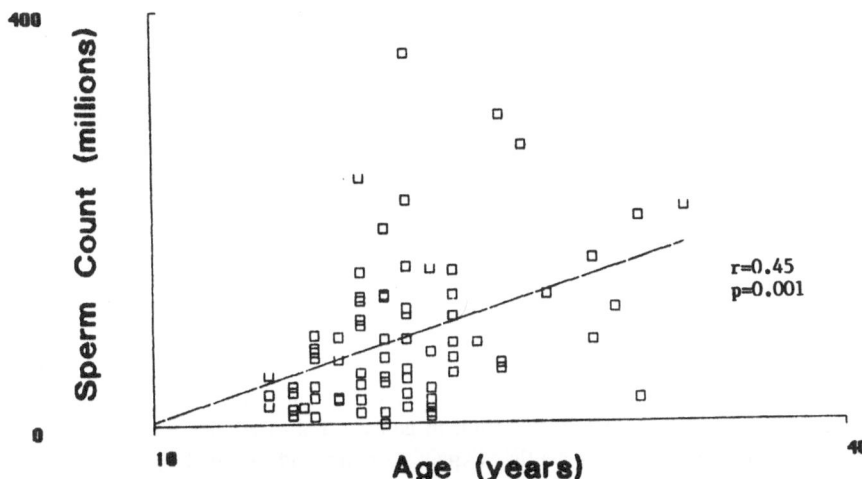

Fig. 6. Correlations between age and total sperm count in patients with β-thalassaemia major

Induction of Spermatogenesis

After gonadotrophin treatment, eight of 21 patients remained azoospermic, but spermatogenesis was induced in 13 patients with hypogonadism or arrested puberty. Of those 13 patients, four had normal spermatogenesis, one had oligospermia (low sperm count) but good motility, and five had oligoasthenospermia (low sperm count and poor sperm motility).

Conclusions

In a recent survey of more than 3000 patients the group studying endocrine complications in nonendocrine diseases of the Italian Endocrine Pediatric Society (SIEDP) found some degree of hypogonadism in 45% of patients, but 55% entered or completed puberty normally [3]. With their assurance of greater longevity, and with the prospect of future marriage, many male thalassaemics wish to know whether they are able to father a child.

Indeed, in our experience, 80 % ot thalassaemics who produce sperm have indicated that they want their sperm stored in a bank because they are interested in having children but concerned about their future fertility. The remaining 20 %, usually aged 16 – 17 years, said that they were too young to consider this aspect.

Essentially, we found that the sperm count was normal in 66 % of patients with β-thalassaemia major and in 80 % with thalassaemia intermedia. Sperm motility was normal in 81 % of patients with β-thalassaemia major and in 70 % with thalassaemia intermedia. Sperm morphology was normal in all patients of both groups.

Our study indicates that follow-up of these patients is important because sperm count may increase with age, and because both sperm count and sperm motility may improve or deteriorate with time.

No correlation was found between sperm count and ferritin concentration, but the majority (86 %)· of patients with thalassaemia major who had serum ferritin levels below 500 ng / ml had abnormal semen analysis.

These data suggest that iron overload per se does not appear to impair spermatogenesis. However, to achieve low serum ferritin levels, intensive, consistent chelation therapy is needed, and this raises the possibility that desferrioxamine may have an adverse effect on sperm production and / or sperm motility. One possible mechanism may be the mild zinc deficiency which chelation can induce. Alternatively, it may be a direct effect of desferrioxamine on the sperm-producing mechanisms [4, 5].

Induction of spermatogenesis was successful in 13 of 21 patients (62 %) with thalassaemia major, four of whom had totally normal sperm production. If one considers that fertile women often conceive even when their partners have substandard semen analyses, these figures are encouraging. In general, thalassaemics who comply with their chelation therapy can usullay expect to enter and complete puberty spontaneously and to be fertile.

References

1. Weatherall DJ, Clegg JB (1981) The thalassaemia syndromes, 3rd edn. Blackwell, Oxford
2. Who Laboratory manual for exmination of human semen human-cervical mucus interation. Press Concern, Singapore, p9
3. Study Group on Endocrine Complications in Thalassaemia (1992) Prevalence of endocrine complications in patients with β-thalassaemia major: an Italian multicenter study (Abstr.) International Mediterranean Conference on Endocrine Disorders in Thalassaemia, May 7–9, Cosenza
4. Netter A, Hartoma R, Nahoul K (1981) Effect of zine administration on plasma testosterone, dihydrotestosterone and sperm count. Arch Androl 7: 69–73
5. De Sanctis V, Katz M, Wonke B, DiPalma N, Mazzotta D, Vullo C (1989) Serum parameters in patients with homozygous β-thalassaemia. Infertility 12: 167–176

Long-term Follow-up of Hypothalamic-Pituitary Axis in Thalassaemic Patients with Secondary Amenorrhoea

R. Chatterjee, M. Katz, and J. B. Porter

Introduction

A wealth of information is available on disturbances of growth and sexual maturation in patients with thalassaemia major [10, 14–18], but four hormonal data are available on secondary amenorrhoea (SA), which is a common sequela in transfusion-dependent thalassaemic patients, occurring in 15–25% of Italian thalassaemic patients [3, 13]. Similar figures are available for the United Kingdom [8].

Objective of Study

We aimed to prospectively evaluate the GnRH-gonadotrophin secretory dynamics in a cohort of 15 menstruating girls with β-thalassaemia major over 10 years to determine whether they sustained progressive damage to the hypothalamic-pit uitary (HP) axis.

Patients

Fifteen thalassaemic girls aged (mean ± SEM) 14.6 ± 0.99 (range: 13.0–16.2) years and five healthy control subjects aged 14.2 ± 0.22 (13.4–16.0) years entered the study. The clinical characteristics of the patients are given in Table 1. The patients had their menarche at the age of 14.2 ± 0.22 (13.4–15.2) years, which was 2 years later than the control subjects 12.2 ± 0.2 (12–13) years. At the initiation of the study, both the patients and the control subjects had regular ovulatory normal menstrual cycles (cycle length = 28 ± 4 days; midluteal progesterone ≥ 30 nmol/l), but all patients became amenorrhoeic within 10 years of their menarche, unlike the control subjects, who continued to menstruate normally. All subjects were euthyroid, and none had significant alteration in her body weight prior to the onset of or during the period of amenorrhoea. The thalassaemic patients received 3 pints of blood every 4–5 weeks and were chelated with 2 g desferrioxamine 5 nights per week plus 2 g with each transfusion. Their overall mean Hb was maintained at approximately 11.5 g% and their transfusion requirement ranged from 120 to 240 units of blood per year. At the beginning of the study all thalassaemic patients had evidence of iron overload with high serum ferritin levels (mean peak serum ferritin

S. Andò et al. (Eds.)
Endocrine Disorders in Thalassemia
© Springer-Verlag Berlin Heidelberg 1995

Table 1. Clinical characteristics of thalassaemic patients with secondary amenorrhoea

Patient number	Chronological age (years)	Heigth (cm)	Weight (kg)	Body mass index (kg/m^2)	Age at menarche (years)	Age at amenorrhoea (years)
1	13.0	142	40	19.8	13.4	23.0
2	16.0	146	44	20.6	14.2	19.2
3	15.2	150	48	21.3	14.0	20.2
4	16.2	152	46	19.9	15.2	22.2
5	13.0	140	42	21.4	14.3	20.4
6	13.6	146	42	19.7	13.8	20.6
7	15.0	150	48	21.3	14.8	19.2
8	14.8	148	46	21.00	14.0	19.6
9	13.6	148	41	18.7	13.0	18.2
10	13.8	142	40	19.8	13.2	20.2
11	14.6	152	48	20.8	14.2	21.4
12	15.2	158	50	20.00	14.5	19.8
13	15.0	150	49	21.9	14.6	20.2
14	14.8	152	52	22.5	14.4	24.2
15	15.2	158	50	20.00	14.6	20.4

Table 2. Haematological parameters in thalassaemic patients: menarche vs amenorrhoea

	At menarche	At onset of amenorrhoea	1 year after onset of amenorrhoea	5–6 years after onset of amenorrhoea
Peak serumferritin (µg/l)	4000.00 ± 100.20 (2000–8000)	3500.00 ± 120.40 (3000–8000)	4000.00 ± 102.40 (3000–8000)	4000.00 ± 100.60 (2000–8000)
Symptomatic organ dysfunction (percentage of patients)	30	30	30	60

= 4000 µg/l), and 30% had evidence of symptomatic organ dysfunction, i.e. cirrhosis, chronic active hepatitis, cardiac arrythmia, imapired glucose tolerance test and diabetes mellitus. At the onset of amenorrhoea and 12–14 months after onset the patients had similar ferritin levels and a similar incidence of organ dysfunction (Table 2). However, 5–6 years after amenorrhoea 60% patients had organ dysfunction despite similar ferritin levels (Table 2).

Methods

The experimental protocol used in this study was approved by the ethical committee of University College and Middlesex Hospital Medical School. Each subject was measured for her heigth (m), weight (kg), and body mass index (BMI in kg/m^2).

The patients had spontaneous and stimulated function of their GnRG-GTH complex assessed at three stages: (a) 18 months to 2 years after their menarche, during both the follicular phase (day 7–8) and the luteal phase (day 22–23) of their menstrual cycles; (b) 12–14 months after the onset of SA; (c) 5–6 years after the onset of SA. The control subjects had similar assessments 18 months to 2 years, 3–4 years and 5–6 years after their menarche. Spontaneous. GTH secretion was assessed by frequent blood sampling to obtain a 12 h ultradian profile. Blood samples (2–3 ml) were drawn at 20-min intervals for 12 h. The sleep-wakefulness period was documented carefully in each subject by observation with the naked eye. Most patients slept between midnight and 6 a.m. After the ultradian profile had been obtained, a standard GnRH test was performed by administering a 100 ug i.v. bolus injection of GnRH and sampling blood at 20-min intervals for 1 h, then at 120 min. Basal samples were assessed for prolactin, TSH, thyroxine and oestradiol (E2) levels. Prolactin, TSH, thyroxine, E2, follicle-stimulating hormone (FSH) and luteinising hormone (LH) were assayed by standard RIA using double-antibody techniques. The sensitivity of both the FSH and the LH assay was 1.6 IU/l and the intra- and interassay CV were less than 10% for all values of FSH and LH. Serum ferritin was measured using an immunoradiometric assay [22]. FSH and LH pulse parameters were analysed statistically using the Pulsar programme [21]. The details of the pulse parameters and values extracted from the GnRH provocative tests are given elsewhere [6, 9]. The Student's paired t-test and the Spearman correlation test were used to analyse the data.

Results and Analysis

All patients had normal bascal prolactin (117.08 ± 1.47 Mu/l), TSH (2.08 ± 0.11 Mu/l) and thyroxine levels (109.44 ± 2.10 nmol/l).

LH Peak Parameters

During the Menstrual Cycle

Table 3 portrays the mean LH peak parameters in the patients during their menstrual cycles and in the control subjects.

Follicular Phase (Day 7–8 of the (cycle)
During the follicular phase, there was little difference in the mean, maxi, PL, PA, ampl and PM values between the patients and the controls. However, the length and the IPI were longer and the peak number was slightly reduced in the patients compared with the controls.

Lutcal Phase (Day 22–23 of the (cycle)
Patients. Although there was little difference in the mean compared with that of the follicular phase, maxi was considerably higher ($p < .001$). Compared with the folli-

Table 3. Peak characteristics of thalassaemic girls during menstrual cycle and 12–24 months after the onset of amenorrhoea and in the control subjects

Group	Mean (IU/l)	Maxi (IU/lO)	Peak no	Ampi (Iu/L)	Length (min)	IPI (min)	PL	PA (IU/l)	PM (IU/l)
LH control (n = 5)									
FP	6.08 ± 0.20	10.90 ± 0.33	7.50 ± 5.60	4.31 ± 0.20	61.83 ± 5.0	88.30 ± 6.80	3.00 ± 0.20	4.20 ± 0.20	8.00 ± 0.31
LP	6.50 ± 0.13	16.30 ± 0.09	7.00 ± 0.77	6.20 ± 0.05	75.60 ± 10.20	99.60 ± 13.50	3.45 ± 0.34	5.90 ± 0.60	9.30 ± 0.60
Patients (n = 5)									
FP	5.98 ± 0.11	10.95 ± 0.30	6.75 ± 0.32	4.90 ± 0.22	70.50 ± 1.80	97.12 ± 3.30	3.50 ± 0.20	4.90 ± 0.20	8.60 ± 0.12
LP	6.40 ± 0.09	16.15 ± 0.20	8.50 ± 0.50	5.30 ± 0.40	59.30 ± 5.80	85.37 ± 9.03	2.80 ± 0.20	5.20 ± 0.5	8.80 ± 0.55
12–14 months post secondary amenorrhoea	4.16 ± 0.19	7.20 ± 0.50	7.70 ± 0.40	2.60 ± 0.13	61.75 ± 4.40	87.25 ± 6.50	3.03 ± 0.20	2.50 ± 0.20	5.40 ± 0.24
FSH controls (n = 5)									
FP	3.80 ± 0.12	6.63 ± 0.08	8.16 ± 0.65	2.20 ± 0.10	58.16 ± 7.13	82.33 ± 7.61	2.77 ± 0.26	2.21 ± 0.14	4.84 ± 0.15
LP	3.51 ± 0.03	6.46 ± 0.15	7.33 ± 0.33	1.81 ± 0.12	58.00 ± 4.14	94.00 ± 5.36	2.84 ± 0.32	1.81 ± 0.17	4.51 ± 0.18
Patients (n = 15)									
FP	3.60 ± 0.07	6.27 ± 0.22	7.50 ± 0.59	1.97 ± 0.08	63.25 ± 6.52	91.00 ± 8.07	2.98 ± 0.24	1.94 ± 0.12	4.51 ± 0.12
LP	3.66 ± 0.12	5.62 ± 0.31	7.62 ± 0.46	1.84 ± 0.07	59.87 ± 4.89	90.25 ± 4.44	2.88 ± 0.24	1.84 ± 0.11	4.51 ± 0.11
12–14 months post secondary amenorrhoea	3.65 ± 0.21	6.65 ± 0.15	8.25 ± 0.12	2.09 ± 0.18	56.25 ± 6.34	79.75 ± 7.53	2.72 ± 0.28	2.05 ± 0.28	4.63 ± 0.21

All values are expressed as mean + SEM.
FP Follicular phase; *LP* lutcal phase.
Controls vs patientx (Spontaneous puberty), not significant

cular phase, the peak number remained unchanged, but the IPI, ampl and length increased. The PL remained unaltered, but PA and PM increased.

Controls. In the luteal phase, the mean and the maxi LH levels were essentially similar to those of the follicular phase. The peak number was higher, while the IPI was shortened. The ampl was increased, while the length was reduced. The PL, PA and PM were also increased. In the lutcal phase, the patients and the controls had similar mean and maxi levels, but the PL, PA, ampl and the PM values were lower

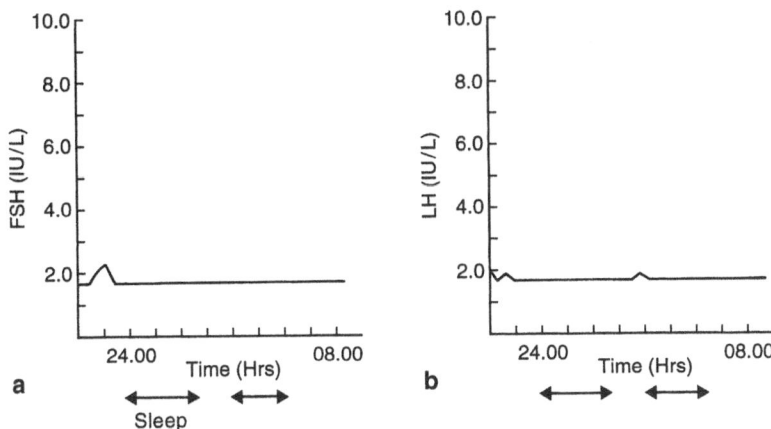

Fig. 1a, b. Apulsatile patterns of (**a**) FSH; (**b**) LH secretion in patient 4. *Bar* represents sleep interval

in the patients than in the controls. Interestingly, the peak number was higher and the IPI was shorter in the patients.

At 12–14 Months After the Conset of Amenorrhoea

It ist evident from Table 3 that, compared with their pre-amenorrhoeic phase, the thalassaemic patients had a marked diminution in their mean, maxi, ampl, PA and PM levels when amenorrhoeic. The length was also diminished, but less strikingly than the aforementioned paramenters. There was, however, no change in the peak number after the onset of amenorrhoea in the patients. Interesting observations were made when sleep-entraind (SE) LH pulses were analysed in the pulsatile patients. In all patients there was a marked increase in the percentage of SE pulses after the onset of amenorrhoea. For instance, in patient 12, the percentage of SE pulses was 61.5% on day 8 and 58.8% on day 22. After amenorrhoea occured, the percentage of SE pulses rose to 70.5%. Similarly, in patient 5, the SE pulse percentage increased from 61.5% on day 8 and 61.5% on day 22 to 78.5% after amenorrhoea occurred. Compared with the controls the SA group had lower mean, maxi, ampl, PA and PM levels, but the other parameters, i.e. peak number, length, PL and IPI, were similar in the two groups. The development of abnormal pulse parameters following the onset of amenorrhoea is indicative of H-P dysfunction.

At 5–6 Years After the Onset of Amenorrhoea

Although patients studied at 12–14 months who had pulse defects all were pulsatile, by 5–6 years 66% of patients had become apulsatile. The remaining 3–4 remained pulsatile but their pulse parameters deteriorated, in that they exhibited multiple pulse defects. Figure 1a and b gives examples of the apulsatile pattern and some of the pulse defects observed in the patients. These findings indicate that H-P

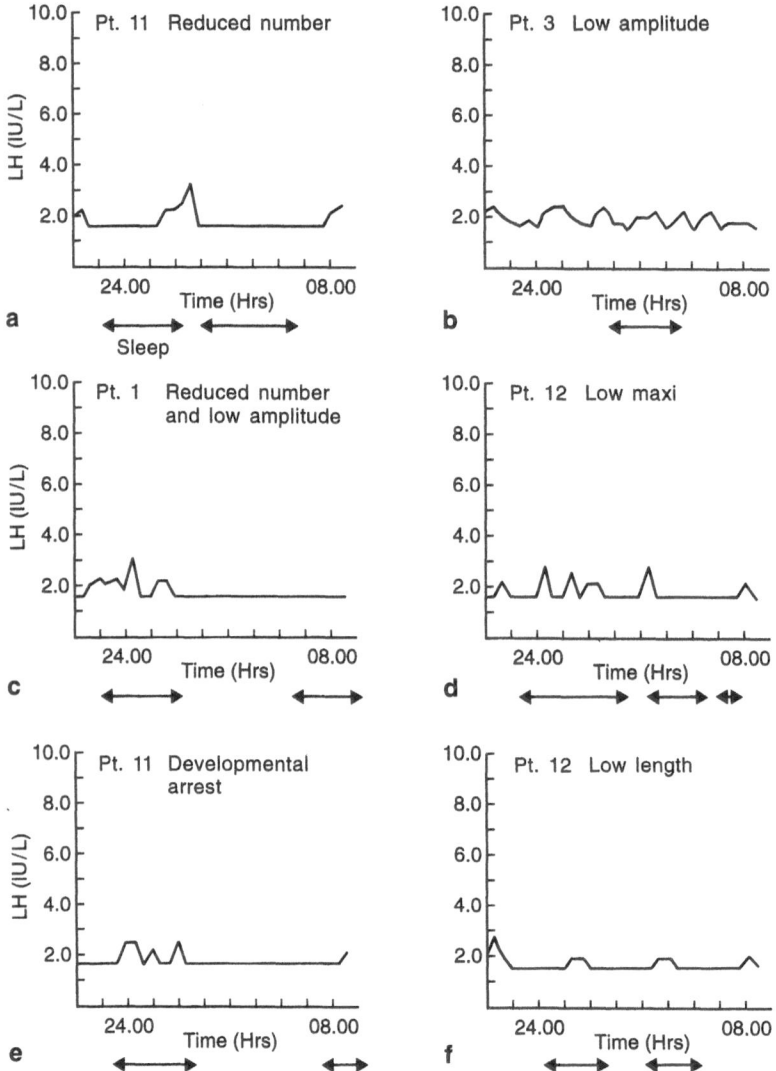

Fig. 2a–f. LH pulse defects in thalassaemic patients with secondary amenorrhoea. (a) Patient 11 had reduced number; (b) patient 3 had reduced amplitude, whereas (c) patient 1 had a combined defect of reduced number and low amplitude; (d) patient 12 had a low maxi; (e) patient 11 had developmental arrest; and (f) patient 12 had low length. *Bars* represent sleep intervals

dysfunction continued in the patients in a progressive fashion, and a specific example of this is given in Fig. 2.

It ist important to note that thalassaemic patients lacked LH pulse variability following amenorrhoea in contrast to their menstrual cycles, when they exhibited variability between their follicular and luteal phases. An example of the lack of LH

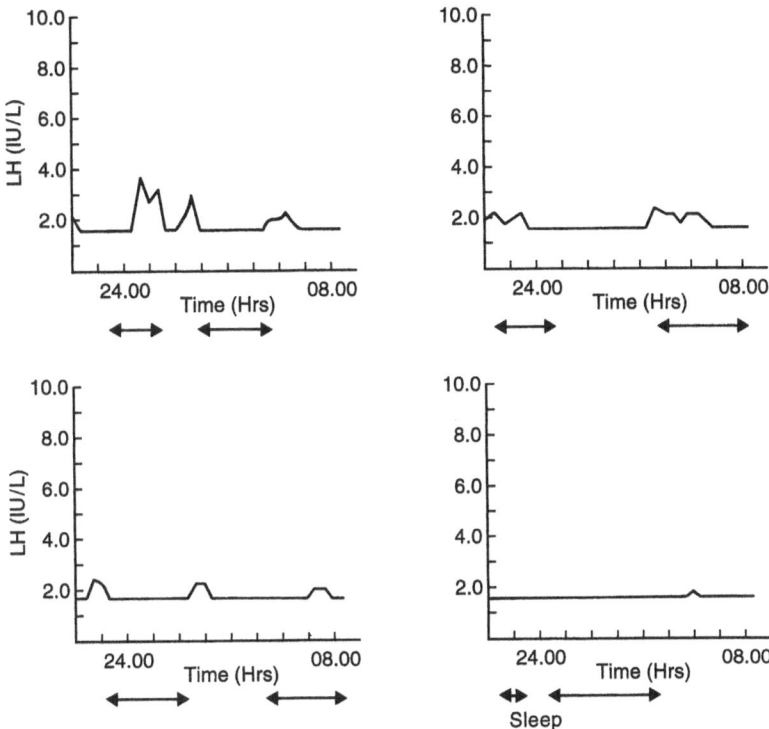

Fig. 3. Progressive deterioration of LH pulses from pulsatile pattern to total apulsatility in a thalassaemic patient (no. 3) at 12–24 months and 5–6 years after the onset of secondary amenorrhoea

peak variability in patients with SA is given in Fig. 3. Moreover, 5–6 years after the onset of SA, this lack of pulse variability became more pronounced, especially in patients who became apulsatile. For instance, all patients who were apulsatile remained so throughout the study period.

FSH Peak Parameters

During the Menstruating Cycle

Follicular Phase (Day 7–8 of the (cycle)

During the follicular phase, the mean, maxi, PA, ampl and PM levels and the peak number were higher in the controls than the patients. By contrast, the IPI and the PL were shorter in the controls.

Luteal Phase (Day 22–23 of the (cycle)

In the patients the mean level was higher, but the maxi was lower than in the follicular phase. The IPI, PL, PA and the ampl were also lower in the luteal phase.

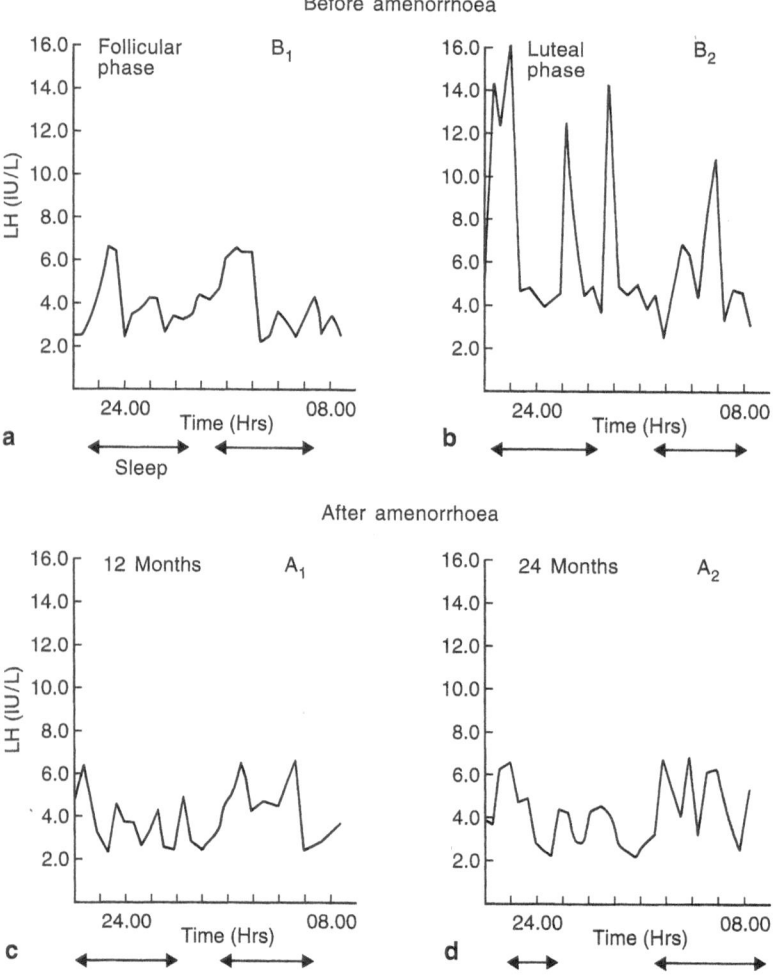

Fig. 4a–d. LH pulse variability in a thalassaemic patient (no. 2) during (**a**) follicular (B1) and (**b**) luteal (B2) phases of menstrual cycle. Note that (**c**) 12 (A1) to (**d**) 24 (A2) months after the onset of secondary amenorrhoea, this patient exhibited good variability of her LH pulses

The difference was statistically different only for the PA values ($p < .001$). There was no difference in the peak number and the PM values between the two phases of the cycle. In the controls the mean was only slightly different compared with that of the follicular phase, but the maxi was considerably higher ($p < .001$). Compared with the follicular phase, the peak number remained unchanged but the IPI increased, as did the ampl, length, PA and PM. The PL remained unaltered.

In the controls the mean, PL, PA, ampl and the peak number were lower, but the maxi was higher and the IPI longer than those of the thalassaemic patients.

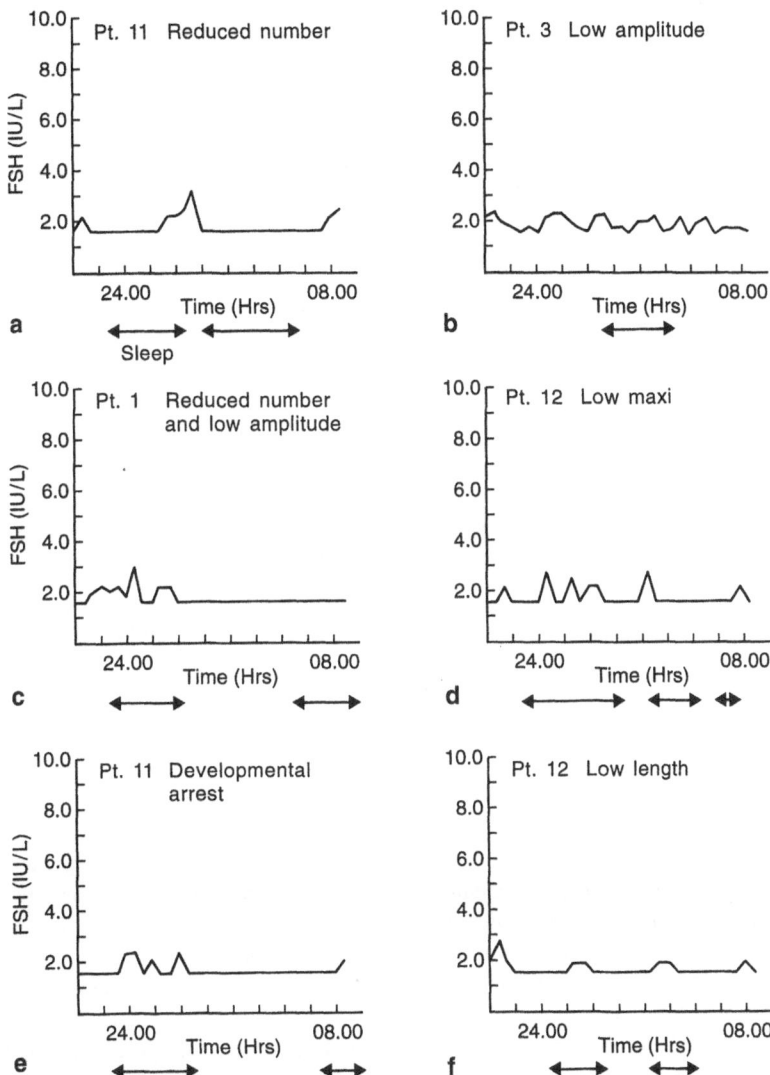

Fig. 5a–f. FSH pulse defects in thalassaemic girls with secondary amenorrhoea. (a) Patient 11 had reduced peak number; (b) patient 3 hat low amplitude; (c) patient 1 hat a combined defect of reduced number and lowamplitude; (d) patient 12 had low maxi; (e) patient 11 had developmental arrest; and (f) patient 12 had short length

At 12–14 Months After the Onset of Amenorrhoea

Twelve to 24 months after the onset of amenorrhoea, patients with SA had similar mean FSH levels but slightly higher maxi levels than during their menstrual cycles. The peak number, ampl, PA, PM were also higher during amenorrhoea, but the length, PL and IPI values were lower. The mean and maxi FSH levels in the

Table 4. FSH and LH response in thalassaemic girls to a 100 µg GnRH bolus before & after the onset of secondary amenorrhoea

Time of study	FSH (IU/l)				LH (IU/l)			
	Basal	Peak	FSH	FAUC	Basal	Peak	LH	LAUC
During menustrual cycles (d7–d8) (n = 15)	2.00 ±0.23	10.20 ±0.22	8.20 ±15.20	822.00 ±15.20	2.20 ±0.24	16.20 ±0.28	14.00 ±0.63	970.00 ±18.00
12–24 months post secondary amenorrhoea	1.20 ±0.22	8.00 ±0.18*	6.20 ±0.21*	740.00 ± 16.00*	2.00 ±0.32	14.20 ±0.80*	12.20 ±0.48*	960.00 ± 16.20*
5–6 years post secondary amenorrhoea								
Pulsatile patients (n = 5)	1.80 ±0.25	6.40 ±0.02	4.60 ±0.08	580.00 ±14.00	2.00 ±0.22	10.20 ±0.22	8.20 ±0.18	840.00 ±10.20
Apulstaile patients (n = 10)	1.62*	3.00 ±0.40*	1.38 ±0.32*	268.00 ± 10.20*	1.66*	2.80 ±0.20*	1.14*	280.00 ±9.20*
Controls (n = 5)	3.80 ±0.20	18.00 ±1.60*	14.20 ±1.38*	1988.00 ± 12.20*	4.60 ±0.24*	20.20 ±1.80*	15.60 ±1.56*	1060.00 ± 16.80*

All values are expressed as mean ± SEM.
Maximum increment FAUC and LAUC are area under the curve for FSH and LH, respectively.
Patients vs controls during their menstrual cycles, $*p < .001$.
Patients: pre vs 12–24 months post secondary amenorrhoea, $*p < .001$.
Pulsatile vs apulsatile patients 5–6 years post secondary amenorrhoea, $*p < .001$.

patients with SA did not change markedly after cessation of menses, whereas for LH pulses both these parameters were markedly reduced after amenorrhoea.

Interestingly, compared with their cycling periods, all patients had a marked rise in the percentage of SE FSH pulses after the onset of amenorrhoea. For instance, in patient 12, the percentage of SE pulses was 57.1% on day 8 and 31.3% on day 22, but 82.3% during amenorrhoea. Similarly, in patient 5, the percentage of SE pulses was 47.4% on day 8, 46.2% on day 22 and 62.5% after the onset of amenorrhoea. These observations regarding sleep entrainment of FSH pulses were similar to those seen in LH pulses in the same patients.

At 5–6 Years After the Onset of Amenorrhoea

Sixty-six percent of patients were apulsatile 5–6 years after the onset of amenorrhoea. The remaining 34% remained pulsatile, but their pulse parameters deteriorated in that they exhibited multiple pulse defects. Figures 1a and 4 give examples of the apulsatile pattern and some of the pulse defects observed in the patients. These findings indicate that H-P dysfunction continued in a progressive fashion.

Gonadotrophin Response to an i.v. Bolus of 100 μg GnRH

During the follicular phase of the menstrual cycles the basal and GnRH-stimulated FSH and LH were lower in the patients than in the control subjects, although the differences were not statistically significant (Table 4). Twelve to 24 months after the onset of amenorrhoea the basal and GnRH-stimulated GTH levels of the patients were markedly and significantly reduced compared with those of their menstrual cycles, and compared to the control subjects. By 5–6 years after the onset of amenorrhoea, the patients had a further reduction in their basal GTH levels and their GTH responses to GnRH. But even those patients with apulsatile GTH profiles responded to a GnRH bolus. However, the apulsatile patients had significantly lower basal and GnRH-stimulated FSH and LH levels than did the pulsatile patients.

Discussion

Retrospective studies suggest that thalassaemic patients with SA have damage to their anterior pituitary glands, consequent to transfusional iron overload, [11, 12, 16]. However, no prospective data are available on the evolution of such damage or on whether there ist hypothalamic involvement in such patients. To our knowledge, this is the first study following thalassaemic girls prospectively from their postmenarcheal menstrual cycles unitl they became amenorrhoeic and then up to 6 years later to determine the degree of their H-P secretory dysfunction.

Our data indicate that, compared with the control subjects, thalassaemic patients had reduced spontaneous GTH secretion during their menstrual cycles. As a group, however, they mimicked the normal subjects, in that they had no GTH pulse defects, and they had low GnRH-stimulated GTH responses. This early evidence of diminished H-P reserves suggested that they were likely to develop secondary amenorrhoea at a later date.This is precisely what was found during their long-term follow-up.

The ampl, frequency and IPI of gonadotrophin pulses are important in regulating ovarian function, including follicular maturation, [2, 20, 23, 24]. And steroidogenesis [1, 23]. Studies by Reame et al. [25] have demonstrated that slow or accelerated pulse frequency and variable amplitude are causally related to cycle disturbances associated with anovulation and may account for hypothalamic amenorrhoea.

The results of this study indicate that thalassaemic girls have progressive deterioration of their H-P function within 2 years after the onset of amenorrhoea. They have multiple pulse defects – a marked diminution in ampl and maxi levels, a significant increase in the percentage of SE pulses and the absence of pulse variability – characteristic of hypothalamic damage.

An increase in SE pulses is physiologic in early puberty [5], but it is also found in recovering anoresctics [4, 19], in whom it represents hypothalamic *developmental arrest*. Since a similar increase in SE pulses is found in thalassaemic patients with SA, it would seem reasonable to propose that they have a derangement in hypothalamic GnRH secretion. This is not the whole story, however, because, unlike patients with anorexia nervosa, they also have primary gonadal insufficiency [7]. Disruption of the gonadal steroid feedback mechanism which invariably accompanies primary gonadal insufficiency must compound the disturbance of GnRH pulsatility. That low plasma oestradiol concentrations play an important role in the genesis of LH pulse abnormalities is inferred from the occurrence of large-amplitude pulses at frequent intervals in patients with *pure* primary ovarian failure [23, 24]. So the combined experience of shorter interpulse intervals between LH pulses with low-amplitude pulses in thalassaemic girls with SA must be a manifestation of both GnRH secretory insufficiency and ovarian damage.

Another characteristic factor which maintains cyclicity of ovarian function in women is the variablility of endogenous. LH rhythm. This is in striking contrast to the stable GnRH secretory pattern of normal adult males. The ovulatory menstrual cycle exhibits considerable variability in pulse characteristics when pasing from the follicular to the luteal phase. This is due to the variable feeback of fluctuating sex steroid levels [26–28]. Similar variability in gonadotrophin pulse patterns, even more marked than in cycling women, was observed by Spratt et al. [28] and Reame et al. [25] to occur in patients with hypothalamic amenorrhoea at 1- to 8-month intervals over a 12- to 24-month period. Variability of LH rhythm is also found in patients recovering from anorexia nervosa [4, 19]. Observations by Kletzky et al. [16] suggest that non thalassaemic patients with secondary amenorrhoea who have little or no GTH fluctuation are likely to have severe hypothalamic-pituitary failure with little chance of spontaneous resumption of menstrual function. If this observation applies equally to thalassaemic female patients with secondary amenorrhoea, the presence or absence of GTH pulse variability could be of great prognostic importance. Their ability to recover menstrual function spontaneously and their potential fertility may depend on whether or not they are found to have GTH pulse variability. We know of no thalassaemic woman who, having developed secondary amenorrhoea, remitted to spontaneous menstrual function. Thus, there seems little point in assessing GTH pulse variability in thalassaemic women with SA, except to differentiate those thalassaemics with secondary amenorrhoea who coincidentally have hypothalamic amenorrhoea and are recovering anorectics, and who could be expected to show marked pulse variability with good prognosis, from the usual thalassaemics with SA in whom the GTH secretory pattern could be expected to be stable with poor prognosis. This concept held true when thalassaemics with SA were re-evaluated 5–6 years after the onset of amenorrhoea. Many patients had become apulsatile, and as a group they had significantly lower GnRH-stimulated GTH levels than during the earlier period of investigation, indicating that despite intensive chelation treatment they had progressive and severe damage to their GnRH-GTH complex.

The exact cause of hypothalamic-pituitary dysfunction in thalassaemic patients with secondary amenorrhoea is unclear. But prior to the onset of amenorrhoea they had normal basal FSH, LH and prolactin levels and they were euthyroid. Moreover, no patient has had an alteration in body weight. Therefore, the pathogenesis of amenorrhoea was likely due either to the chronic ill health associated with thalassaemia or to its treatment, i.e. transfusion iron overload or desferrioxamine toxicity. The former seems more likely, since patients in the study group were heavily iron over-loaded and many of them had symptomatic organ dysfunction.

Our results have many important clinical implications. Firstly, with irrefutable evidence that H-P damage exists well before the onset of amenorrhoea, all efforts should be made to ensure compliance with treatment from an early age rather than at the onset of amenorrhoea. Vigilant follow-up after thalassaemic girls have experienced menarche is essential, since they are vulnerable to develop secondary amenorrhoea even if they have had intensive transfusion and chelation therapy. Secondary amenorrhoea carries on ominous prognosis with little chance of spontaneous recovery. But since patients have potentially intact ovaries, albeit with diminished ovarian reserve, ovulation can usually be induced artificially by HMG treatment in patients keen on pregnancy, especially during their early years of amenorrhoea. Attempts to achieve pregnancy should not be delayted in couples with a stable relationship unless cogent reasons exist for doing so.

References

1. Backstom LT, McNeilly AS, Leask RM, Baird DT (1982) Pulsatile secretion of LH, FSH, prolactin, oestradiol and progesterone during the human menstrual cycle. Clin Endocrinol (Oxf) 17: 29
2. Baird, DT (1983) Factors regulating the growth of the pre-ovulatory follicle in the sheep and the human. J Reprod Fertil 69: 343
3. Borgna-Pignatti C, De Stefano PL, Zonta MS, Vullo C, De Sanctis V, Melevendi C, Naselli A, Masera G, Terzoli S, Gabutti V, Piga A (1985) Growth and sexual maturation in thalassaemia major. J Paediatr 106: 150
4. Boyar RM, Finkelstein JW, Roffwarg HP, Kapen S, Weitzman E, Hellman L (1972) Synchronization of augmented luteinizing hormone secretion with sleep during puberty. N Engl J Med 287: 582
5. Boyar RM, Finkelstein JW, Hoffwarg H, Kapen S, Weitzman ED, Hellman L (1973) Twenty-four hour luteinising hormone and follicle-stimulating hormone secretory patterns in gonadal dysgenesis. J Clin Endocrinol Metab 37: 521
6. Chatterjee R (1992) Ultradian gonadotrophin profiles in patients with beta-thalassaemia major. PhD thesis, University of London
7. Chatterjee R, Katz M, Wonke B (1989) Secondary amenorrhoea in patients with thalassaemia major (Abstr 346). 3rd World Congress on Fertility and Sterility, Marrakesh
8. Chatterjee R, Katz M, Wonke B, Porter JB (1992) Long-term follow-up of hypothalamic-pituitary axis in patients with secondary amenorrhoea (Abstr 10). International Mediterranean Conference on Endocrine Disorders in Thalassaemia, May 7–9, Cosenza
9. Chatterjee R, Katz M, Cox TF, Porter JB (1993) Prospective study of the hypothalamic-pituitary axis in thalassaemic patients who developed secondary amenorrhoea. Clin Endocrinol (Oxf) 39: 287–296
10. Chatterjee R, Katz M, Cox TF, Bantock HM (1993) Evaluation of growth hormone in thalassaemic boys with failed puberty: spontaneous versus provocative test. Eur J Paediatr 152: 721–726
11. Costin G, Logut MD, Hyman CB, Ortega JA (1979) Endocrine abnormalities in thalassaemia major. Am J Dis Child 133: 497
12. De Sanctis V, Vullo C, Katz M, Wonke B, Hoffbrand AV, Bagni B (1988) Hypothalamic-pituitary-gonadal axis in thalassemic patients with secondary amenorrhoea. Obstet Gynecol 72: 643
13. De Sanctis V, Pintor C, Andò S et al. (1992) Prevalance of endocrine complications in patients with β-thalassaemia major: an Italian multicenter study (Abstr 1). International Mediterranean Conference on Endocrine Disorders in Thalassaemia, May 7–9, Cosenza

14. Erlandson ME, Brilliant R, Smith CH (1964) Comparison of sixty-six patients with thalassaemia major and thirteen patients with thalassaemia intermedia including growth, development, maturation and prognosis. Ann NY Acad Sci 119: 727
15. Johnston FE, Hertzog KP, Malina RM (1966) Longitudinal growth in thalassaemia major. Am J Dis Child 122: 396
16. Kletzky OA, Costin G, Marrs RP, Bernstein G, March CM, Mishell DR Jr (1979) Gonadotrophin insufficiency in thalassaemia major. J Clin Endocrinol Metab 48: 901
17. Kuo B, Zaino E, Roginsky MS (1968) Endocrine function in thalassaemia major. J Clin Endocrinol Metab 28: 805
18. Lassman MD, O'Brian RT, Pearson HA, Wise JK, Donabedian RK, Felig R, Genel M (1974) Endocrine evaluation in thalassaemia major. Ann NY Acad Sci 232: 226
19. Marshal JC, Kelch RP (1979) Low-dose pulsatile gonadotrophin-releasing hormone in anorexia nervosa: a model of human pubertal development. J Clin Endocrinol Metab 49: 712
20. McNatty KP, Gibb M, Dobson C, Thurley DC (1981) Evidence that changes inluteinsing hormone secretion regulate the growth of the pre-ovulatroy follicle in the ewe. J Endocrinol 90: 375
21. Merriam GR, Watcher KW (1982) Algorithms for the study of episodic hormone secretion. Am J Physiol 243: E310
22. Miles LE, Lipseitz DA, Bieber CP, Cook JD (1974) Measurement of serum ferritin by a two-site immunradiometric assay. Ann Biochem 61: 209
23. Peluso JJ, Gruenberg ML, Steger RW (1984) Regulation of ovarian follicular growth and steroidogenesis by low-amplitude LH pulses. Am J Physiol 15: R184
24. Pohl CR, Knobil E (1982) The role of the central nervous system in the control of ovarian function in higher primates. Annu Rev Physiol 44: 583–593
25. Reame N, Sauder SE, Case GD, Kelch RP, Marshall JC (1985) Pulsatile gonadotrophin secretion in hypothalamic amenorrhoea: evidence that reduced frequency of gonadotrophin-releasing hormone secretion is the mechanism of persistent anovulation. J. Clin Endocrinol Metab 61: 851
26. Rebar RW, Yen SSW (1979) Endocrine rhythms in gonadotrophins and ovarian steroids with reference to reproductive processes. In: Krieger DT (ed) Endocrine rhythms. Raven, New York, p 259 (Comprehensive endocrinology Series)
27. Santen RJ, Bardin CW (1973) Episodic luteinising hormone secretion in man: pulse analysis, clinical interpretation, physiologic mechanisms. J Clin Invest 52: 2617
28. Spratt DI, Carr DB, Merriam GR, Scully RE, Rao N, Crowley WF (1987) the spectrum of abnormal patterns of gonadotrophin-releasing hormone secretion in men with idiopathic hypogonadotrophic hypogonadism: clinical and laboratory correlations. J Clin Endocrinol Metab 64: 283

Abnormal Bone Metabolism in Thalassemia

P. J. Giardina, R. Schneider, M. Lesser, B. Simmons, A. Rodriguez,
J. Gertner, M. New, and M. W. Hilgartner

Introduction

Historically, homozygous beta-thalassemia major has been associated with marked
osseous changes, originally described by Cooley et al. in 1927 [1]. The pathogenesis of the abnormal bony changes has been ascribed to the underlying massive
ineffective erythropoiesis and erythroid expansion of medullary bone, and the subsequent thinning of cortical bone, as well as metabolic and endocrine dysfunction
secondary to hemochromatosis [2, 3]. Concurrent osteopenia results in frequent
pathological fractures and premature epiphyseal fusion [4, 5].

In recent years, the administration of regular transfusion thereapy to maintain a
near normal hemoglobin level has resulted in partial suppression of the ineffective
erythropoiesis and has prevented or partially improved the bony abnormalities [6].
Nevertheless, radiographically significant osteopenia, cortical thinning, and trabeculation remain [7].

.Osteopenia has traditionally been evaluated by standard radiographs which allow
for only a qualitative analysis. More recently, densitometry allows for a quantitative
measure of bone mineral content and is a valuable tool for assessing risk of fracture
and for monitoning treatment response of bone mineral content in various pathological states [8]. Various densitometry modalities exist, including single- or dual-photon absorptiometry (SPA, DPX), quantitative computed tomography (CT), or
dual energy X-ray absorptiometry (DEXA). Normative data of bone mineral density
(BMD) using these modalities have been documented for males and females in
childhood, adolescence, and adulthood by several authors [9–12].

We have measured bone mineral content in grams of ash per cm^2 by densitometry
(BMD) using DPX and DEXA and report our findings in thalassemia major subjects maintained on regular transfusion and iron chelation therapy. We report the
occurrence of fractures in these subjects over the past 15 years, since the institution
of "hyper"-transfusion regimens in our program. We compare thalassemic BMD of
the lumbar vertebrae (L2–4) to reference data of previously described age-matched
controls and determine the mean standard deviation scores (Z scores) for spinal
BMD in thalassemia major male and female children, adolescents, and adult
subjects.

S. Andò et al. (Eds.)
Endocrine Disorders in Thalassemia
© Springer-Verlag Berlin Heidelberg 1995

Methods

Subjects with Thalassemia Major

All thalassemia major subjects were recruited from the thalassemia transfusion clinic in the Division of Pediatric Hematology at The New York Hospital-Cornell Medical Center after giving informed consent. The 69 thalassemia subjects ranged from 3 to 37 years of age; 29 were male and 40 were female. A total of 99 BMD studies were performed, each subject having one or more serial studies performed over a 5-year study period.

All subjects are maintained on a "hyper"-transfusion program to achieve a pretransfusion hemoglobin level greater than 10.5 gm/dl. However, the oldest subjects, above the age of 20 at the time of the study, had been historically maintained on a "low"-transfusion program at hemoglobin levels of 7–8 gm/dl and were escalated in the mid 1970's to a "hyper"-transfusion program. Subjects under the age of 19 at the time of the study had been maintained on a "hyper"-transfusion program since infancy or early childhood.

All subjects are maintained on an iron chelation program with desferrioxamine (Desferal) administered subcutaneously via an 8-h infusion each day. The dosage varies from 40 to 60 mg/kg body wt. and is recommended to be used 5 nights each week.

Table 1. Incidence of fractures among New York Hospital-Cornell Medical Center thalassemia population

	Prior to 1976 [5]	1977–1991
No. of patients	25/75 (33%)	22/110 (20%)
Age range (years)	3–31	2–37
Median age (years)	12	13
Mean age (years)	12.8 ± 7.0	15.6 ± 8.4
No. of fractures	47	22
Fracture sites		
Leg bone	31	7
Vertebrae	5	12
Hip	0	3
Fusion	7	0

Table 2. Correlations between spinal bone mineral density and other variables in thalassemia major

Group	No. of patients	Age (years)	Height (cm)	Weigth (kg)	BMI
< 19 years	70	0.76	0.78	0.78	0.49
p =		0.0001	0.0001	0.0001	0.0001
> 20 years	29	0.03	0.52	0.53	0.23
p =		0.889	0.003	0.003	0.227

Control Subjects

The control subjects were chosen from spinal BMD reference data from previously described Caucasian, nonthalassemic, age-matched children, adolescents, and adults obtained by DPX [11–13].

Physical Measurements

Height was measured to the nearest 0.1 cm on a mall-mounted stadiometer. Weight in kilograms with clothes, but without shoes, was measured on a balance scale.

Record Review of Skeletal Fractures

Medical clinic records of 110 thalassemia subjects followed up at NYH-CMC from 1976 to 1991 were reviewed for documentation of skeletal fractures.

Lumbar Spine Densitometry Measurements

Bone mineral content densitometry (BMD) of the lumbar portions of the spine (L2–4) was performed in 66 studies with a dual-photon densitometer (DPX, Novo Lab 22), which records the absorption of a dual-photon beam emission from two independent sources and is highly reproducible. DPX measures both cortical and trabecular bone density. Thirty-six spinal BMD studies were performed with DEXA (Lunar). DEXA was done on a LUNAR DPX-L dual-energy radiographic densitometer using a fast scan made with 1.68 mm collimation, sample size 1.2 x 1.2 mm, and a current of 3000 UA. the current software is version 1.3 Y. Software versions were updated as indicated by the company.

Statistical Analysis

Multiple regression analysis was performed using spinal BMD as the dependent variable and sex, age, weight, and body mass index at the time of testing as independent variables. The subjects were separated for analysis into two groups, those less than 19 years and those greater than 20 years of age.

Results

In Table 1 the occurrence of bone fractures in thalassemic subjects followed between 1977 to 1991 is only slightly lower than that previously reported in 1976 [5]. Currently, fewer long bone fractures and more vertebral compression fractures have occurred, with no episodes of premature epiphysial fusion.

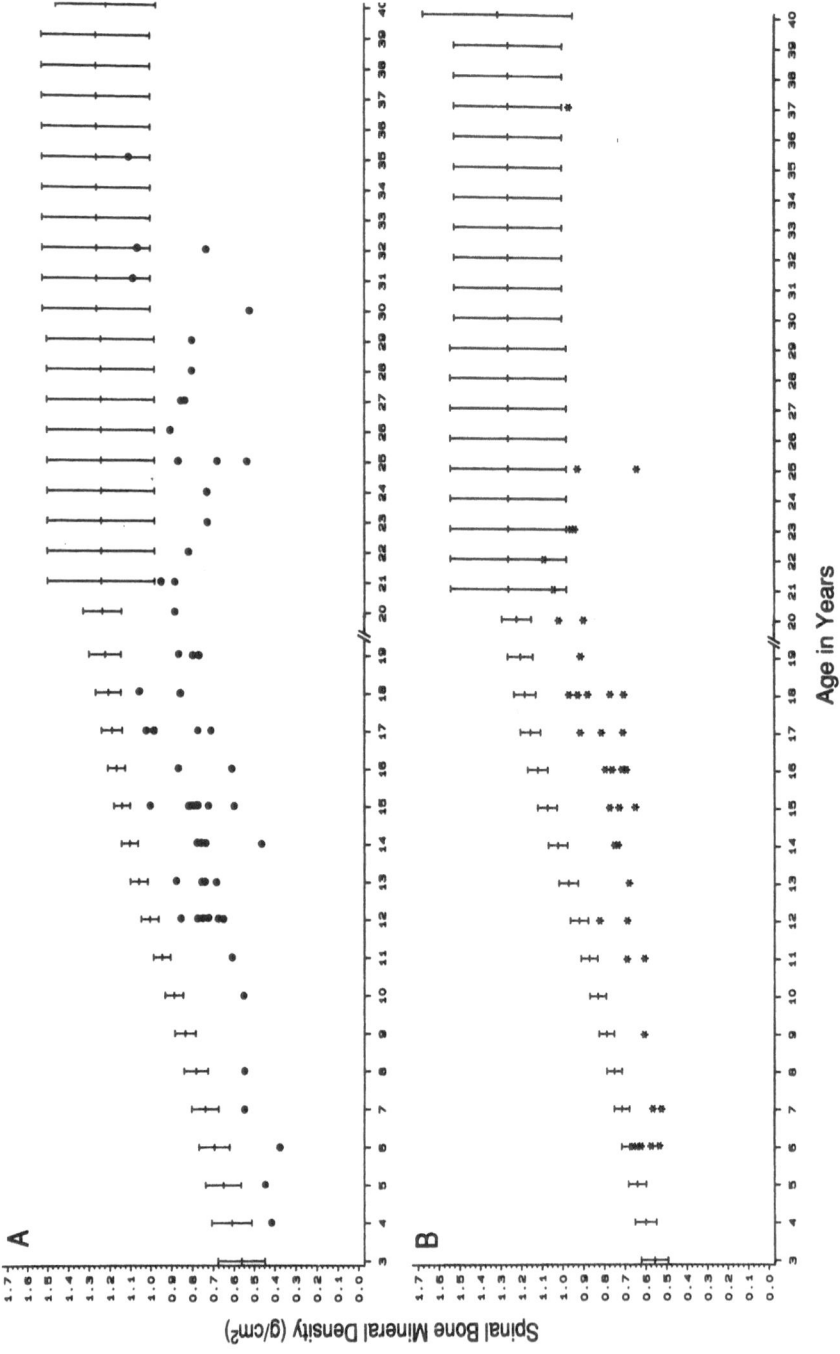

Fig. 1 A, B. Forty female thalassemia major subjects (*A*, ●) ranging from 3 to 35 years of age and 29 male subjects (*B*, *) ranging from 6 to 37 years of age have BMD measures lower than the standard reference controls, but which increase with age

Table 3. Mean bone mineral density in thalassemia major children, adolescents, and adults

Sex	No. of BMD studies	Mean age (years)	Mean BMD (grams of ash/cm^2)
M	12	8.9 ± 3.1	0.63 ± 0.1
F	20	9.9 ± 3.2	0.63 ± 0.1
M	18	15.0 ± 4.4	0.81 ± 0.1
F	19	15.5 ± 3.3	0.80 ± 0.1
M	11	25.9 ± 1.9	0.96 ± 0.1
F	22	25.6 ± 5.4	0.85 ± 0.2

Table 2 demonstrates that age, height, weight, and body mass index are highly correlated with spinal BMD content in thalassemic children, adolescents, and young adults. The degree of correlation of the variables is most evident in the younger age-groups, those younger than 19 years, when weight, height, and body mass index as well as spinal BMD are changing with age. Regression analysis demonstrates that when all of these variables are considered together, body weight is significantly related to spinal BMD.

The spinal BMD measures of male and female thalassemic subjects are lower than the normal reference controls but change with age, increasing through the second decade, as do the controls (Fig. 1 A, B).

In Table 3 the spinal BMD mean ± standard error of the mean (SEM) in male and female thalassemia major subject groups demonstrates that there are no apparent sex differences in the spinal BMD of the children and adolescent subjects, whereas the adult male subjects have significantly higher levels ($p < 0.05$) than those of female subjects.

The Z score, i.e., the number of standard deviations from the normal mean for each subjects, is calculated, and the scatter correlation plots of the thalassemia major children and adolescent subjects demonstrate that Z scores change with age. The mean Z score of those subjects younger than 19 years is –12.5 ± 5.6 (range –0.8 to –30.0 S.D.). The majority of adult subjects also have BMD less than 2.0 S.D. below the norm for age. However, the mean Z score of the adult subjects above 20 years of age remains more stable than those seen in the younger thalassemic subjects at –3.4 ± 1.8 S.D. (range –1.2 to –8.8 S.D.).

Discussion

Abnormal bone metabolism in thalassemia has been attributed to the expansion of the erythron mass owing to the massive ineffective erythropoietic process and the chronic hypoxia associated with the severe anemia [1, 2]. However, other mechanisms such as local trace metal imbalance, excess iron, or the secondary effects of hemochromatosis with variable multiorgan endocrine dysfunction may also contribute to local bone formation [14, 15].

In normal bone formation, bone is constantly being remodeled, i.e., resorbed and reformed by osteoclast and osteoblast activity. Bone turnover is regulated by the responsiveness of osteoclasts to parathyroid hormone, glucocorticoids, vitamin D, sex steroids, insulin, prostaglandins, cytokines, and growth factors. Trace metals are essential and function as cofactors in reactions for bone production and mineralization. Iron excess is also known to inhibit pyrophosphatase, and precipitates pyrophosphate crystals as well as influencing osteoblastic numbers and activity [14].

There have been reports of impaired parathyroid reserve and reduced parathyroid hormone levels in thalassemia causing impaired calcium exchange [19]. Vitamin D, which stimulates intestinal absorption of calcium and regulates osteoblastic function, may be deficient. Impaired skeletal growth has been associated with impaired thyroid function, and subnormal somatomedin activity occurs [20, 21]. The deranged functions of the hypothalamic-pituitary-gonadal axis contributes to alterations in gonadotropin pulse secretion, gonadal failure, and growth retardation, with normal and subnormal growth hormone secretion and growth hormone release [22].

The classical skeletal manifestations of thalassemia initially described by Cooley et al. and subsequently reported by others have been historically defined by clinical and radiographic findings [1, 2]. Widening of the medullary cavity leads to disproportions of the diaphysis and a characteristic "squared" appearance of long bones, referred to as tubulation [16]. Cortical thinning results from the inability of new bone formation to keep pace with resorption. The diploic space of the skull becomes widened and provides the characteristic "hair-on-end" appearance [2]. The vertical vertebral striations or the appearance of fine or coarse cystic spaces within the cortex of long bones results from the coarsening of the trabecular pattern of bone and a dropout of all but the mechanically most necessary trabeculae [16]. Skeletal dysmaturation has been radiographically associated with premature fusion of the humeral and/or femoral epiphyses. Prior to "hyper"-transfusion therapy, Curarrino and Erlandson reported that premature epiphyseal fusion occurred in 23% of thalassemic patients over the age of 10 years [4].

In recent years, the amelioration of these skeletal deformities has been ascribed to normalizing transfused hemoglobin levels [17]. However, radiographic evidence of osteopenia persists and pathological fractures continue to occur, despite modern transfusion and chelation practice. Papageorgiou's review of thalassemia patients maintained on "hyper"-transfusion and chelation regimens demonstrated that 91% developed osteopenia, 70% had cortical thinning, and 37% had increased trabeculation of the spine [7].

A review of the fracture history of our patients treated with "hyper"-transfusion and chelation therapy since 1977 has revealed that although the types of fractures have changed, with fewer long bone fractures and more vertebral compression fractures, their occurrence only decreased from 33% to 20% and premature epiphyseal fusions did not develop.

The persistence of osteopenia and fractures prompted our assessment of bone mineral content, which can be determined by a variety of densitometry modalities. Single-photon absorptiometry and dual-photon absorptiometry use photons; these units of electromagnetic energy form a radionuclide source of gamma energy that is absorbed at different rates in bone and soft tissue. Dual-energy X-ray absorptiometry (DEXA) uses photons generated by an X-ray tube at two energy levels and has less radiation exposure of $1-3$ mrads, as compared with DPX at 15 mrads.

As seen in reference controls, thalassemic spinal BMD is highly correlated with age, height, weight, and body mass index. Body weight is most highly correlated with BMD in subjects less than 19 years of age ($p < 0.001$) and greater than 20 years ($p < 0.003$), suggesting that spinal BMD is more responsive to load-bearing reflected by body weight than to chronological age. Spinal BMD of thalassemia subjects also changes with age, increasing through the second decade. However, nearly all thalassemic subjects attain spinal BMD far below that of age-matched reference controls, and nearly all the adult subjects have BMD below $1.0 \, g/cm^2$, which increases their risk of fractures.

The Z scores of the thalassemic subjects younger than 19 years with a mean of -12.5 ± 5.6 worsen with age, which may reflect the degree of "hyper"-transfusion therapy, progressive transfusional iron load, the degree of compliance with chelation therapy, progressive transfusional iron load, the degree of compliance with chelation therapy, or complications of chelation [23]. Historically, the adolescent thalassemic years are subject to progressive transfusional hemochromatosis with multiorgan endocrine dysfunction. Our thalassemic subjects have variable degrees of hypothyroidism, parathyroid dysfunction, diabetes mellitus, and poor or delayed, or even reversal of, sexual maturation, which may contribute to their significantly abnormal Z scores. The scatter correlation plot of Z scores for those subjects greater than 20 years of age with a mean of -3.4 ± 1.85 S.D. over time remain more stable than those for the younger subjects. The fact that subjects older than 20 years have better Z scores than younger subjects suggests that bone mineral content improves with maturation; however, these older subjects may represent a selective population of thalassemics who have survived into their third decade salvaged by current management strategies.

No sex differences are documented in the growing child and adolescent thalassemic subjects. However, adult female thalassemic subjects have significantly lower ($p < 0.05$) spinal BMD than adult male subjects. The occurrence of delayed or absent menarche in nearly 40 % of our female subjects, and transient estrogen production with secondary amenorrhea in almost 30 %, may account for their decreased spinal BMD as adults. Densitometry can play a significant role in the evaluation of supplemental estrogen, calcium, and vitamin therapies in thalassemic subjects, as well is in monitoring and preventing osteoporosis and fracture risk.

It is extremely important to point out the limitations of this study. First, ideally we should have used reference controls of similar ethnic background. Second, our sample size is small and can only be the beginning of a reference range for thalassemic children and adults. Third, the subjects selection may be biased toward symptomatic subjects who were eager to participate.

In summary, it appears that abnormal bone mineral content, as measured by spinal BMD in grams of ash per cm^2, is present in nearly all thalassemia major subjects, regardless of "hyper"-transfusion and chelation therapy begun in early childhood or during adolescence and young adulthood. Abnormal thalassemic BMD undoubtedly reflects bone pathology of multiple etiologies, including the local effects of unsuppressed bone marrow expansion and iron toxicity, as well as secondary endocrinopathies and possibly trace metal imbalance and vitamin deficiencies. Further longitudinal studies should be performed to address these multiple variables, and serial BMD can be a useful guide to address bone pathology and to monitor treatment strategies and their efficacy.

References

1. Cooley TB, Witwer ER, Lee P (1927) Anemia in children with splenomegaly and peculiar changes in the bones. Am J Dis Child 34: 347–363
2. Caffey I (1975) Cooley's anemia: a review of the roentgenographic findings in skeleton. Am JR 78: 381–391
3. Canale VC (1974) Beta thalassemia: a clinical review. Pediatr Ann 3: 6–30
4. Currarino G, Erlandson ME (1964) Premature fusion of epiphyses in Cooley's anemia, Radiology 83: (4): 656–664
5. Dines DM, Canale VC, Arnold WD (1976) Fractures in thalassemia. J Bone Joint Surg [Am] 58: 662–666
6. Piomelli S, Danoff SJ, Becker MH et al. (1969) Prevention of bone malformations and cardiomegaly in Cooley's anemia by early hypertransfusion regimen. Ann NY Acad Sci 165: 427–436
7. Papageorgiou O, Papanastasiou DA, Beratis NG (1991) Scoliosis in β-thalassemia. Pediatrics 88: 341–345
8. Cummings SR (1987) Bone mineral densitometry (Health and Public Policy Committee). Ann Intern Med 107: 932–936
9. Ponder SW, McCormick DP, Fawcett D et al. (1990) Spinal bone mineral density in children aged 5.00 through 11.99 years. Am J Dis Child 144: 1346–1348
10. Glastre C, Braillon P, David L et al. (1990) Measurement of bone mineral content of the lumbar spine by dual energy X-ray absorptiometry in normal children: correlation with growth parameters. J. Clin Endocrinol Metab 70: 1330–1333
11. Thomas KA, Cook SD, Bennett JT et al. (1991) Femoral neck and lumbar spine bone mineral densities in a normal population 3–20 years of age. J Pediatr Orthop 11: 48–58
12. Mazess RB, Barden HS, Ettinger M et al. (1987) Spine and femur density using dual-photon absorptiometry in US white women. Bone Miner 2: 211–219
13. Mazess RB, Barden HS, Drinka PJ (1987) Influence of age and body weight on spine and femur bone mineral density in US white men. J Bone Miner Res 5: 645–651
14. DeVernejoul MC, Pointillart A, Golenzer CC et al. (1984) Effects of iron overload on bone remodeling in pigs. Am J Pathol 166: 377
15. Diamond T, Stiel D, Posen S (1989) Osteoporosis in hemochromatosis: iron excess, gonadal deficiency of other factors. Ann Intern Med 110: 430–436
16. Aksoy M, Camli N, Dincol K, Erdem S, Dincol G (1973) On the problem of 'rib-within-a-rib' appearance in thalassemia intermedia. Radiol Clin Biol 42: 126–133
17. Kattamis C, Touliators N, Haidas S et al. (1970) Growth of children with thalassemia: effect of different transfusion regimens. Arch Dis Child 45: 502
18. Giardina PJ, Grady RW, Ehlers KH et al. (1990) Current therapy of Cooley's anemia: a decade of experience with subcutaneous desferrioxamine. Ann NY Acad Sci 162: 275–285
19. Gabrielle O (1971) Hypoparathyroidism associated with thalassemia. South Med J 64: 115–116
20. Flynn DM, Fairney A, Jackson D et al. (1976) Hormonal changes in thalassemia major. Arch Dis Child 51: 828–836
21. Saenger P, Schwartz E, Markenson AL et al. (1980) Depressed serum somatomedin activity in beta thalassemia. J Pediatr 96: 214–218
22. Modell B, Berdoukas V (eds) (1984) Growth, puberty and endocrinopathy. In: The clinical approach to thalassemia. Grune and Stratton, London PP 175–197
23. DeVirgillis S, Congia M, Frau F et al. (1988) Deferoxamine-induced growth retardation in patients with thalassemia major. J Pediatr 113: 661–669

Bone Mineral Content
by Single- and Dual-Photon Absorptiometry
in Thalassemic Patients

M.-H. Goni, V. Markussis, and G. Tolis

Introduction

β-Thalassemia major (β-TM) is a hereditary, fatal hemolytic anemia relatively common in Mediterranean countries. Chronic hypoxia secondary to anemia, extramedullary hematopoiesis, hepatosplenomegaly, osteoporosis, cardiac failure, and increased susceptibility to infections contribute to the mortality and morbidity associated with the disease. Hypertransfusion therapy, although it has dramatically increased the duration and quality of life of thalassemic patients, invariably leads to chronic iron overload, despite chelation, resulting in cardiomyopathy, hepatic cirrhosis, hyperpigmentation and multiple endocrine abnormalities, the most common being hypogonadotrophic hypogonadism.

Osteopenia is an important problem in β-thalassemia, as it leads to numerous pathologic fractures which, in one fifth of the patients, are multiple and recurrent and may cause severe limb deformities and functional impairment [1]. Red marrow overstimulation and hyperplasia, due to ineffective erythropoiesis, producing widening of the medullary space and cortical thinning appears to be the major pathogenetic factor for osteoporosis in thalassemic patients. Increased iron deposition on bone resulting in abnormal bone turnover, low plasma vitamin D concentrations, diabetes, and, more rarely, secondary hypoparathyroidism or hypothyroidism owing to iron overload may constitute additional mechanisms.

On the other hand, the beneficial effect of sex steroids on bone is well established. Men with delayed puberty and hypogonadism of any cause and women with prolonged amenorrhea at any stage of their reproductive life or during the first postmenopausal years exhibit a substantial decrease in bone mass which is ameliorated by the institution of hormone replacement [2, 3]. Young male and female thalassemic patients are prone to develop low bone mass because of the nature of their disease as well as because of deficiency of gonadal steroids. However, despite the well-known severity and implications of the problem, the exact incidence of osteoporosis in thalassemic hypogonadal populations has not been sufficiently studied at present; moreover, the possible result of prolonged hormone replacement therapy on their bone mass is unknown.

Therefore, this study was designed in order to assess bone mineral density (BMD) at different sites of the appendicular and axial skeleton in a population suffering from homozygous β-thalassemia and particularly in hypogonadal thalassemic patients, both untreated and receiving hormone replacement for varying time periods.

S. Andò et al. (Eds.)
Endocrine Disorders in Thalassemia
© Springer-Verlag Berlin Heidelberg 1995

Patients and Methods

A total of 143 thalassemic patients were studied. They all received transfusions every 20–30 days to maintain their hemoglobin concentrations between 9 and 10 g/dl, and they were chelated 5–6 times a week with the iron-chelating agent desferrioxamine by means of a subcutaneous pump. Patients with clinical hypothyroidism, classic GH deficiency, abnormal serum calcium levels, clinically overt diabetes mellitus, and active liver disease were excluded from the study. Pubertal status was assessed on the basis of Tanner staging, LHRH testing (100 μg i. v.) and testosterone/E_2 levels. Bone age was determined from a left-hand X-ray.

Analytically, there were 59 male thalassemic patients aged 20.7 ± 5.4 (13–38) years; their BMI was 20.1 ± 3.3 kg/m^2 and ferritin levels were 2911 ± 525 ng/ml. Seven male patients had progressed into puberty, although they exhibited a relative sexual maturational delay. Forty-five patients were considered to have primary hypogonadism, while another seven were classified as having secondary hypogonadism. Thirty-one of the 59 male patients had delayed bone age compared with their chronological age. In addition, 84 female thalassemic patients were studied; their BMI was 20.2 ± 2.5 kg/m^2 and ferritin levels were 3793 ± 2241 ng/ml. Seven patients were menstruating, though they were oligomenorrheic, 49 patients had primary amenorrhea, and 28 presented with secondary amenorrhea. Forty female patients were also delayed in bone age. The majority of the patients (male and female) had received hormone replacement therapy for varying time periods in the form of cyclical conjugated estrogens p. o. (0.625 mg) with medroxyprogesterone acetate (5 mg) or a low-dose triphasic contraceptive (female patients), or in the form of testosterone undecanoate (40 mg p. o. 2 or 3 times a day) or testosterone enanthate 250 mg in monthly i. m. injections (male patients). Accordingly, all the patients were assessed to determine the years of hormonal impact on the skeleton by adding the duration of physiologic gonadal function to the duration of hormone replacement.

The bone mineral density (BMD) of the mid radius was determined by 125 I-single-photon absorptiometry (Norland Crp, Fort Atkinson, WI). Scans were obtained from the junction of the proxima two thirds and distral one third of the nondominant radius, a site that contains approximately 95 % cortical bone [4]. Bone density of the distal radius was also measured by single-photon absorptiometry (SPA) at a site corresponding to a distance of 8 mm between radius and ulna. This site is thought to contain 60 % cortical and 40 % trabecular bone [4]. BMD of the lumbar spine was determined in the second through fourth lumbar vertebrae (L_{2-4}) by dual-photon absorptiometry (Lunar Radiation, Madison, WI). This technique measures approximately 50 % trabecular bone [4].

Values are expressed as mean $\pm$ SD. Results were analyzed using the unpaired Student's t-test and Pearson's correlation coefficient.

Results

The bone mineral density (BMD) was globally reduced in our β-TM population. BMD was measured in 32/59 male β-TM patients with SPA, at both distal and proximal sites of the radius, and in 27/59 with dual-photon absorptiometry (DPA) of the lumbar spine, at the L_{2-4} level. SPA was used in 47/84 female patients and DPA in the rest of them. Results are expressed as bone mineral content per surface area (g/cm^2) and also as percentage of expected values in age- and sex-matched controls.

The distal radial BMD with SPA in male patients was (mean ± SD) 0.84 ± 0.16 g/cm^2 ($67.0 \pm 13.6\%$ of expected) and the proximal SPA values were 0.99 ± 0.22 g/cm^2 ($64.4 \pm 14.6\%$). Lumbar BMD with DPA was 0.75 ± 0.15 g/cm^2 ($69.6 \pm 12.8\%$). In female patients distal SPA values were 0.72 ± 0.13 g/cm^2 ($66.5 \pm 12.5\%$ of expected), proximal SPA values were 0.96 ± 0.16 g/cm^2 ($72.3 \pm 11.8\%$), and lumbar DPA values were 0.79 ± 0.17 g/cm^2 ($69.6 \pm 13.8\%$). The loss of more than 20% of the BMD compared with the matched controls is considered significant; 48/59 (81%) of the male patients and 63/84 (75%) of the female patients were below the 80% of expected BMD threshold (Fig. 1a and b).

Consequently, patients were stratified according to their exposure to gonadal steroids (either physiologically or as hormone replacement for hypogonadism) in to four groups: 0–1 years, 2–4 years, 5–8 years, and > 9 years. When BMD (as percent of expected values) was compared in these groups, no significant differences were found in either male of female patients. However, in our female patients BMD measured by DPA correlated positively with the duration of exposure to gonadal steroids ($r = 0.37$, $p < 0.02$) and BMD measured with SPA at distal radius (as percent of expected) correlated negatively with duration of hypogonadism ($r = -0.31$, $p < 0.05$).

Other correlations in male patients included distal radial BMD (SPA) with height ($r = 0.36$, $p < 0.03$), proximal radial BMD (SPA) with age ($r = 0.48$, $p < 0.01$) and weight ($r = 0.43$, $p < 0.01$), and lumbar BMD (DPA) with body mass index ($r = 0.44$, $p < 0.02$) and Tanner stage ($r = 0.38$, $p < 0.05$). In female patients, distal radial BMD (SPA) correlated with bone age ($r = 0.38$, $p < 0.02$), proximal radial BMD (SPA) with body mass index ($r = 0.29$, $p < 0.05$), and lumbar BMD (DPA) with Tanner stage ($r = 0.47$, $p < 0.01$) and bone age ($r = 0.37$, $p < 0.05$) No correlations were found between BMD and ferritin levels in our thalassemic population.

Discussion

Our study showed that adolescent and young adult, male and female, thalassemic patients exhibit a significant loss of cortical and trabecular bone, as determined by SPA and DPA measurements of the radius and the lumbar spine. BMD values lower than 80% of age- and sex-matched controls were found in 81% of the male patients and 75% ot the female patients; by any method used, this represents a loss of more than 1 SD (which is asociated with a 50–100% increase in fracture risk) [5].

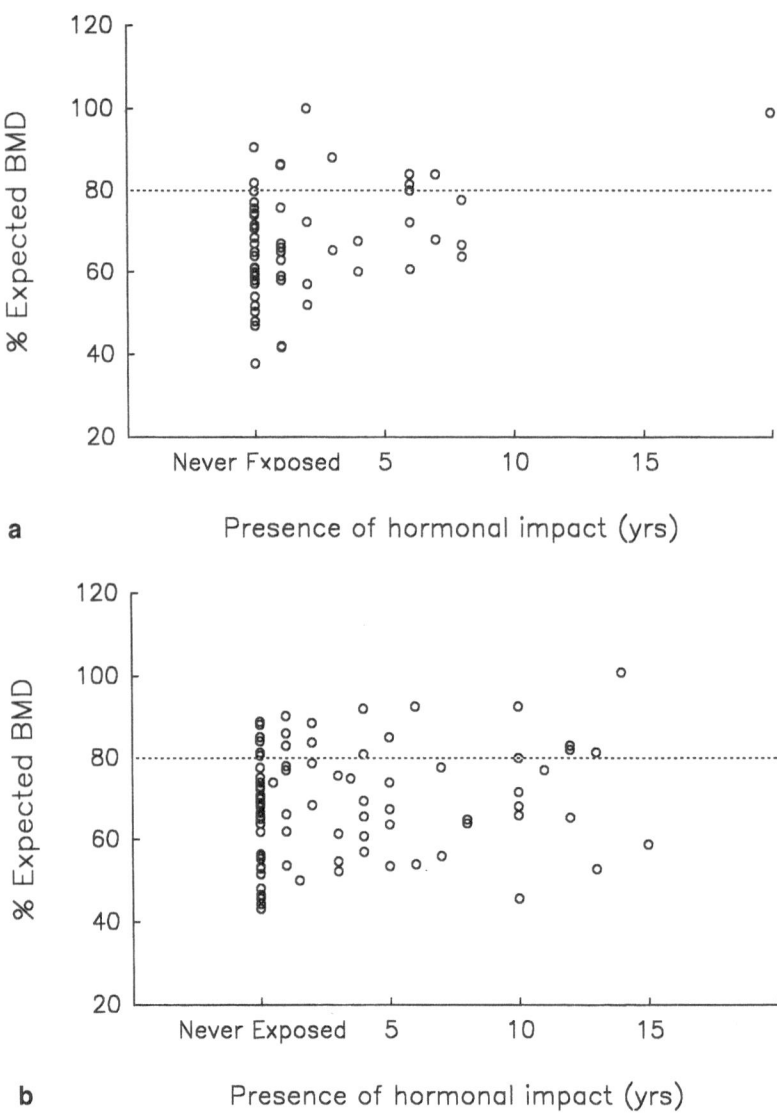

Fig. 1a, b. Bone mineral density (BMD) in male (*a*) and female (*b*) thalassemic patients, according to years of exposure to gonadal steroids (physiologically or as hormone replacement). BMD was measured either at the lumbar spine (L_{2-4}) with DPA or at the distal radius with SPA and is expressed as percent of expected BMD in matched controls. Values lower than 80% of the expected are thought to represent significant bone loss

Previous studies have shown a linear increase in bone mass accumulation up to the years of young adulthood, with an acceleration during puberty [6]. This was verified in our study, since BMD measurements correlated positively with Tanner stage in both male and female thalassemic patients. However, after a certain chronologic age BMD seems to plateau at suboptimal values. The deleterious effect of an even transient delay in gonadal maturation upon bone accretion is well known, and the timing of puberty has been documented as an important determinant of final bone density [2]. In our population, puberty was either absent or delayed, and even in those who received hormone replacement BMD increased but did not reach normal values. This is in accordance with recent studies in hypogonadal patients whose bone mineral density failed to normalize despite their achievement of skeletal maturity after undergoing replacement therapy [2, 3]. However, replacement therapy with sex steroids in our thalassemic patients may have been suboptimal, in terms of either intestinal absorption of oral testosterone formulations or patients' compliance to the prescribed dose. In addition, although hormone regimens needed to produce pubertal maturation are known, information is lacking on optimal doses for long-term promotion of normal bone mass [3]. Moreover, bone disease in β-thalassemia is certain to be multifactorial [1]. In our female population, BMD measurements correlated negatively with duration of amenorrhea and positively with cummulative hormone presence (either physiologic or substituted). It may be that prolonged hormone replacement therapy is needed before significant improvement in BMD becomes obvious.

Further studies are probably required in large numbers of thalassemic patients for long periods of time to determine whether bone mineral density can be normalized by more prolonged therapy and if the increased fracture risk can be ameliorated, in view of the multifactorial etiology of the osteopenia, with earlier institution of treatment.

References

1. Exarchou E, Politou C, Vretou E, Pasparakis D, Madessis G, Caramerou A (1984) Fractures and epiphyseal deformities in beta-thalassemia. Clin Orthop 189: 229–233
2. Finkelstein JS, Neer RM, Biller BMK, Crawford JD, Klibanski A (1992) Osteopenia in men with a history of delayed puberty. N Engl J Med 326: 600–604
3. Emans JS, Grace E, Hoffer Fa, Gundberg C, Ravnikar V, Woods ER (1990) Estrogen deficiency in adolescents and young adults: impact on bone mineral content and effects of estrogen replacement therapy. Obstet Gynecol 76: 585–592
4. Genant HK, Faulkner KG Gluer CC (1991) Measurement of bone mineral density: current status. Am J Med 91 [Suppl 5B]: 49–53
5. Johnston CC, Slemenda CW, Melton LJ III (1991) Clinical use of bone densitometry. N Engl J Med 324: 1105–1109
6. Bonjour JP, Theintz G, Buchs B, Slosman D, Rizzoli R (1991) Critical years and stages of puberty for spinal and femoral bone mass accumulation during adolescence. J Clin Endocrinol Metab 73: 555–563

Osteopenia in Thalassemic Patients with Primary and Secondary Amenorrhea

B. Bagni, V. De Sanctis, I. Bagni, A. R. Cavallini, G. Bonaccorsi, and C. Vullo

Recent reports demonstrate a reduction of bone mineral content on the distal radius in thalassemic patients over the age of 9 years [1–3]. The possibility of accurately measuring bone density at the level of the lumbar spine and femur has significantly improved the sensitivity of measurements in thalassemic patients with primary and secondary amenorrhea, using double X-ray absorptiometry (DXA), to investigate the incidence of osteopenia and its correlation with age, duration of amenorrhea, and biochemical markers of calcium metabolism.

Materials and Methods

In order to evaluate the incidence of induced osteoporosis in thalassemic patients we measured the bone density at the spine and femur using DXA in a group of patients with primary and secondary amenorrhea. The bone density was correlated with the duration of amenorrhea, age, and the biochemical markers of bone methabolism.

We studied 56 thalassemic patients aged 13–40 years (mean age 23 years): 34 patients had primary and 22 secondary amenorrhea for a duration of 1–21 years (mean 6 years), due in all to reduced secretion of gonadotropins (LH and FSH) [4–6].

All the patients were transfused regularly with packed red cells at a pretransfusional hemoglobin level of 5–6 g/dl from the 1960s, gradually increasing to 11.5–12 g/dl in the early 1980s, and at 10.5 g/dl from 1985 to the present. Chelation therapy with desferrioxamine mesylate (Desferal, Ciba-Geigy) was given by the subcutaneous route from 1979 on. The dose and the number of administrations per week were gradually modified during the course of the years. The chelation therapy was carried out during the night (10–12 h), initially at a dose of 20 mg/kg/d on alternating nights, later increased to 5–6 times a week. From 1985 on the dose was increased to 40–45 mg/kg/d [7,8].

The compliance with chelation therapy varied among patients with cardiac insufficiency, thyroid and parathyroid pathology and insulin-dependent diabetes. Patients receiving treatment with calcium, vitamin D, diuretics, and antiepileptics and those who had been estroprogestinic therapy in the past 6 months (four patients) were excluded.

S. Andò et al. (Eds.)
Endocrine Disorders in Thalassemia
© Springer-Verlag Berlin Heidelberg 1995

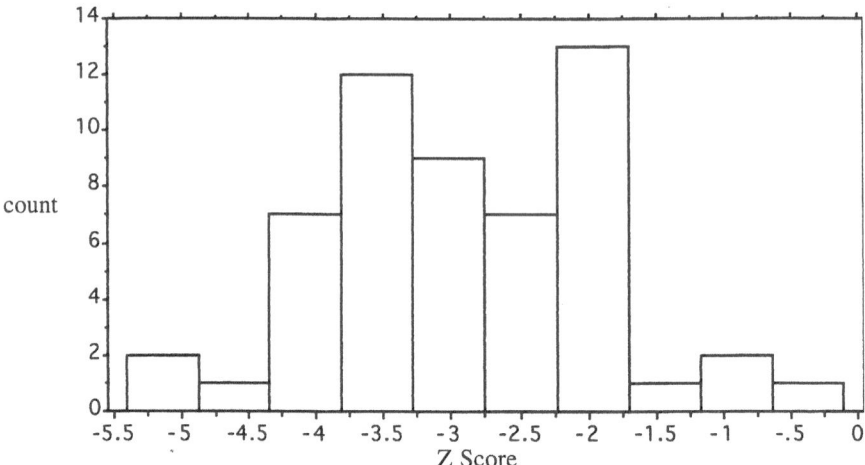

Fig. 1. Spinal BMD Z score distribution in the population of amenorrheic thalassemic patients

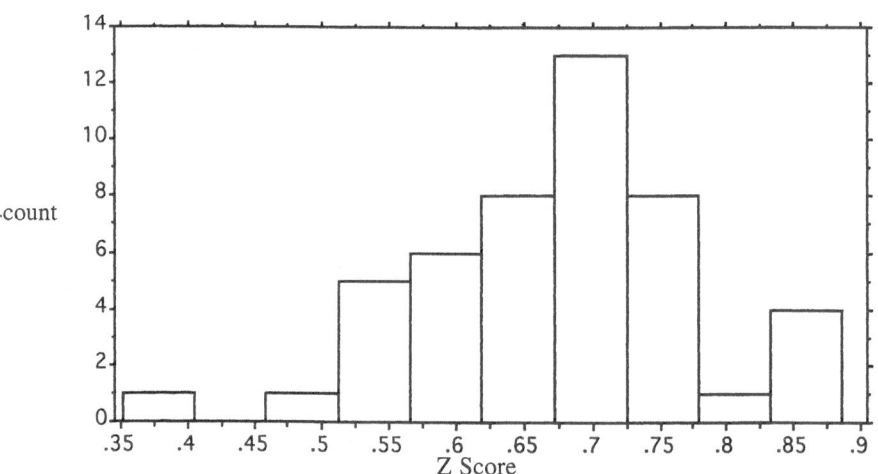

Fig. 2. Femoral (neck) BMD Z score distribution in the population of amenorrheic thalassemic patients

For every patient the following data were recorded: weight, height, duration of amenorrhea, serum transaminase, calcium, phosphate, and creatinine, bone Gla proteinparathyroid, hormone, and iron deposits, evaluated by the measurement of serum ferritin.

Bone density was measured at the lumbar spine, from L2 to L4, and at the femur (Trocanter, Word triangle, global) using an X-ray DXA device with a precision error of 1% in vivo; The Z score was used to evaluate the degree of osteopenia.

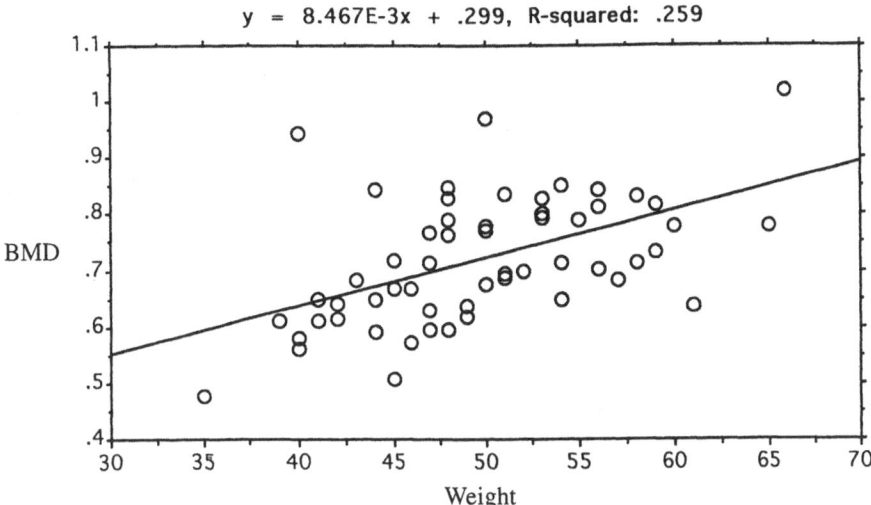

Fig. 3. Spinal BMD vs. weight in amenorrheic thalassemic patients

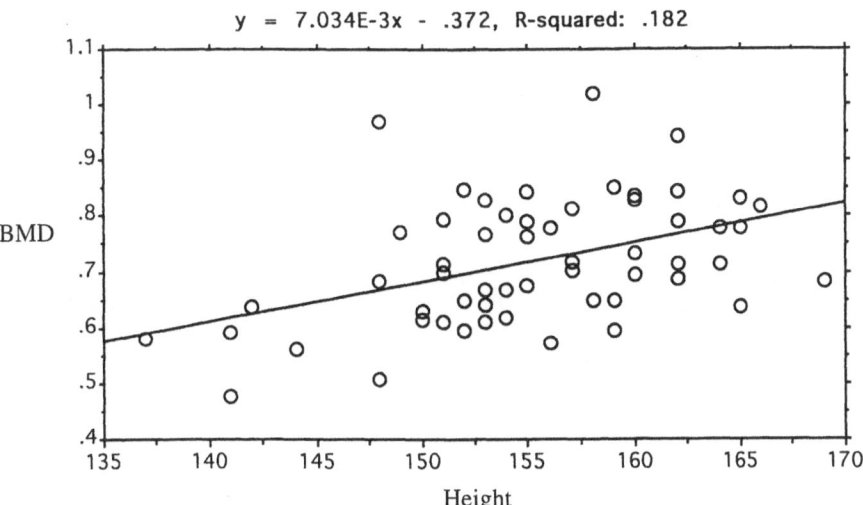

Fig. 4. Spinal BMD vs. height in amenorrheic thalassemic patients

Results

In Figs. 1 and 2 are sumarized the distribution of Z scorė of BMD at the spine and of BMD at the femur, obtained by DXA. The control range used was supplied from the manufacturer and checked by us with a small population survey. A Z score of less than −2 was found in 81 % of the patients. A very significant correlation between bone density at the spine and weight and height was observed (Figs. 3 and 4); in the

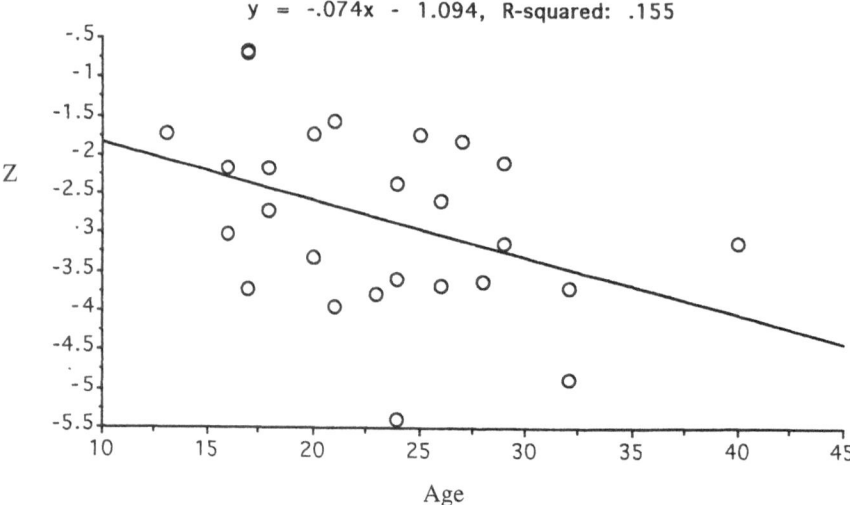

Fig. 5. Spinal BMD Z score vs. age in secondary amenorrhea

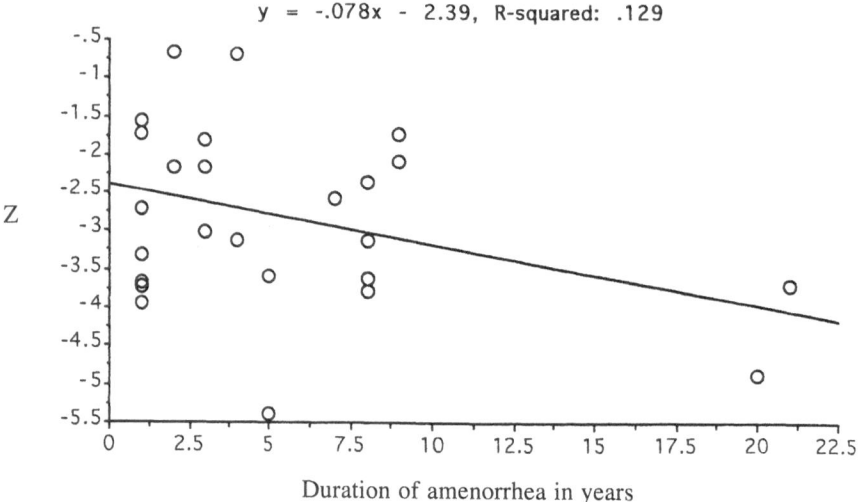

Fig. 6. Spinal BMD Z score vs. duration of amenorrhea

patients with secondary amenorrhea there was a weak correlation between Z score, age, and the duration of amenorrhea (Figs. 5 and 6). No statistical correlation was observed between bone density and calcium parathyroid hormone and serum ferritin.

Discussion

The results of our study show an incidence of osteopenia of 81 % (Z score less than −2 at the spine) in the thalassemic patients with primary and secondary amenorrhea. Bone density is also below the normal range at the femur. The degree of osteopenia appears to be less evident in patients with a greater body mass index and with recent development of amenorrhea.

It is difficult to assess the relative importance of the simple factor which can cause the osteopenia, and it is possible that it is not the same in all subjects. This could be related to differences in the duration of the transfusional regimen at low hemoglobin level, duration of amenorrhea, the presence or absence of chronic liver diseases, or other complications which may affect bone metabolism.

References

1. Bagni B, De Sanctis V (1986) Densitometria ossea in pazienti talassemiche con regolari cicli mestruali, amenorrea primaria e secondaria. In: De Sanctis V (ed) La maturazione sessuale nella beta-talassemia major. International Meeting, Sept 12–13, Ferrara, pp 149–158
2. Ramazzina E, Nardi A, Luisetto G (1986) Metabolismo minerale e scheletrico nell beta-talassemia omozigote. In: De Sanctis V (ed) La maturazione sessuale nella beta-talassemia major. International Meeting, Sept 12–13, Ferrara, pp 249–263
3. Iolascon G, Ronca D, Crusco R (1989) La densitometria ossea computerizzata nel follow-up della malattia di Cooley. 15th National Congress of A.I.E.OP, April 26–30, Turin
4. Drinkwater B, Nilson K, Chesnut TCH (1984) Bone mineral content of amenorrheic and eumenorrheic athletes. N Engl J Med 311: 277–281
5. Cann CE, Martin MC, Genant HK (1984) Decreased spinal mineral content in amenorrheic women. J 251: 626–629
6. De Sanctis V, Atti G, Lucci M (1980) Endocrine assessment of hypogonadism in patients affected by thalassemia major. Clin Lab 10: 663–670
7. Propper RD, Button LN, Nathan DG (1980) New approaches to the transfusion management of thalassemia. Blood 55: 55–61
8. Aldouri MA, Wonker B, Hoffbrand AV (1987) Iron state and hepatic disease in patients with thalassaemia major, treated with long-term subcutaneous desferrioxamine. J Clin Pathol 40: 1353–1359

Imaging, Ultrastructural Aspects, and Trace Elements in the Thalassemic Condrodystrophy

E. Giuzio, M. Bria, F. Romeo, M. Misasi, and C. Brancati

Introduction

Bone diseases are often present in subjects affected by thalassemia major and appear with different pathological features during growth or adult age [1]. According to anatomopathological standards, the group of bone diseases observed during growth are characterized by cartilaginous lesions due mainly to both premature and asymmetrical fusion of the metaphyseal cartilage, while those observed in adults are expressed by skeleteal lesions [2–4]. In this paper we evaluate the lesions involving both the distal metaphysis of the femur and the proximal metaphysis of the tibia in thalassemic children between 8 and 11 years of age.

Material and Method

The patients were routinely transfused with concentrates of washed and filtered red blood cells following a regimen which in the past 5 years allowed us to obtain mean pretransfusional levels of hemoglobin of 10.3 ± 0.75 g/dl. The mean value for serum ferritin was 2557 ± 1595 ng/dl (180–8503). All of the patients received iron-chelating therapy by slow subcutaneous infusion of desferrioxamine (Desferal) 5–6 times weekly at an average dose of 50 mg/kg/day.

All patients in the study underwent radiological, histological, and chemical examinations. We generally carried out radiological investigations by X-ray, computerized transverse cross-sectional tomography, nuclear magnetic resonance imaging, and Tc_{99} scintigraphy.

The histological survey allowed us to observe the anatomopathological aspects of the samples taken from the condrodystrophic areas. Chemical examination was realized by EDAX (energy dispersive analysis X-ray); this technique showed the atomic composition of the sample.

Results

In thalassemic patients suffering from thalassemic condrodystrophy (TC) a macrolacunar aspect of the knee metaphysis can be shown, radiologically. This lesion

S. Andò et al. (Eds.)
Endocrine Disorders in Thalassemia
© Springer-Verlag Berlin Heidelberg 1995

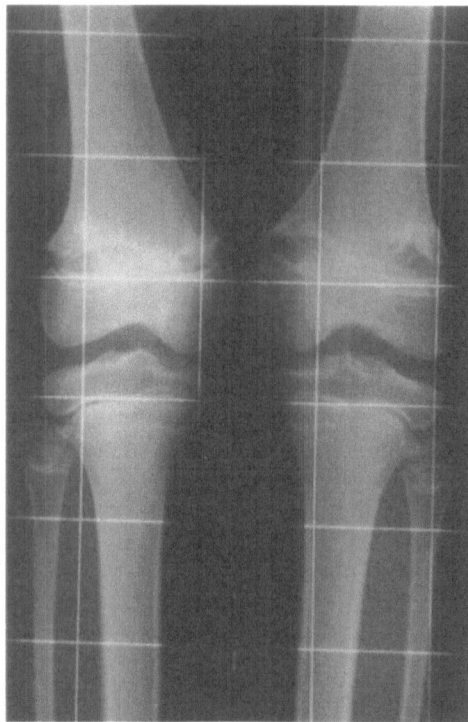

Fig. 1. Radiological aspect of thalassemic condrodystrophie unfused cartilage has, at both its femoral and its tibial levels, a microlacunar aspect with enlarged metadiaphyseal slope, giving to the femoral metaphysis an "owl-eyed" aspect, emphasized by a thin sclerotic edge

gives the femoral metaphysis an "owl-eye" aspect, emphasized by a thin sclerotic edge [5–8]. (Fig. 1).

Sometimes the prevalence of either sclerotic or erosive phenomena can be observed, as well as large erosions with remarkable trabecular longitudinal septa, in both the femur and the tibia (Fig. 2). During growth, the metaphyses of the knee exhibiting a high cell-proliferative rate, are greatly involved. It should be noted that these lesions may also characterize different areas, such as the distal metaphysis of the tibia or the distal metaphysis of the ulna. Transverse cross-section computerized tomography reveals a deep erosion of the metaphysis of the femoral condyles (Fig. 3). This clearly shows that the calcification front has been upset at the epiphysis-metadiaphysis interface. This is caused by a non-calcified fibrous-like tissue, which involves the whole condyle structure. The larger part of the lesion falls within the larger area of the calcification front, and the heterogeneity of the lesion is clearly shown by the presence of calcified tissue areas through a fibrous-like tissue. The lesion decreases as we move from the calcification front. Magnetic resonance imaging also shows the presence of pathological tissue along the calcification front both on transverse and sagittal sections. Using technetium 99m, an element which reveals the metabolic-functional activity of the lesion by fixing the phosphates, the femoral condrodystrophic areas appear to have less uptake in comparison with other, more fertile areas. These data show that the lesions are characterized by slowed calcium turnover.

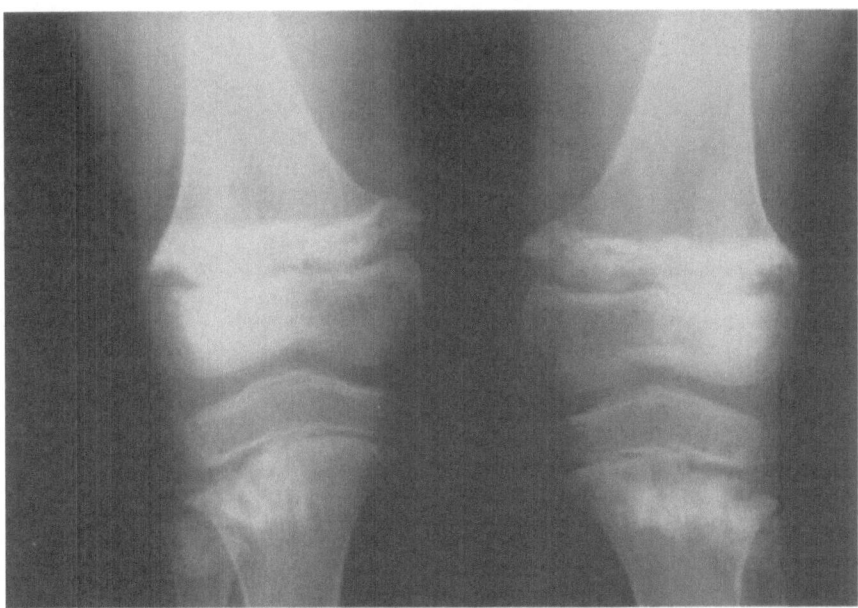

Fig. 2. Particular aspect of thalassemic condrodystrophy caused by the presence of a large erosion in the femoral metaphysis, with large trabecular longitudinal septa

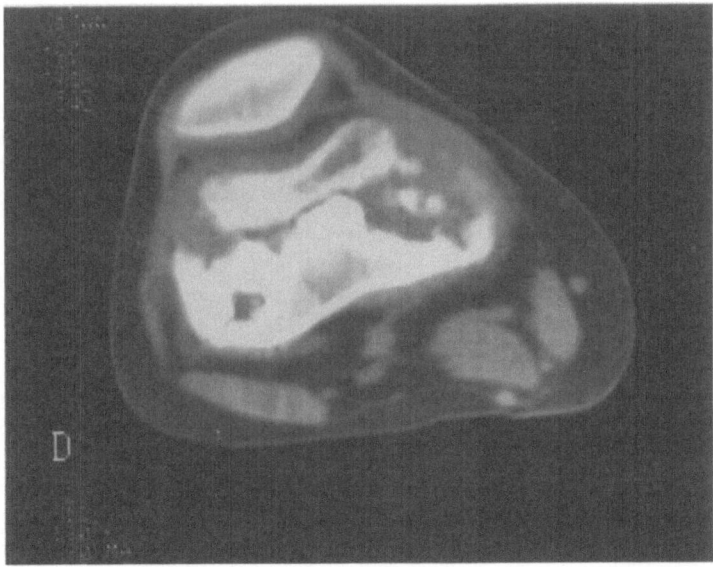

Fig. 3. Computerized tomography on a transverse cross section shows a deep erosion of the metaphysis in the area between the epiphysis and the metadiaphysis. This aspect is caused by a noncalcified fibrous-like tissue which invades the calcification front at the epiphysis-metadiaphysis interface

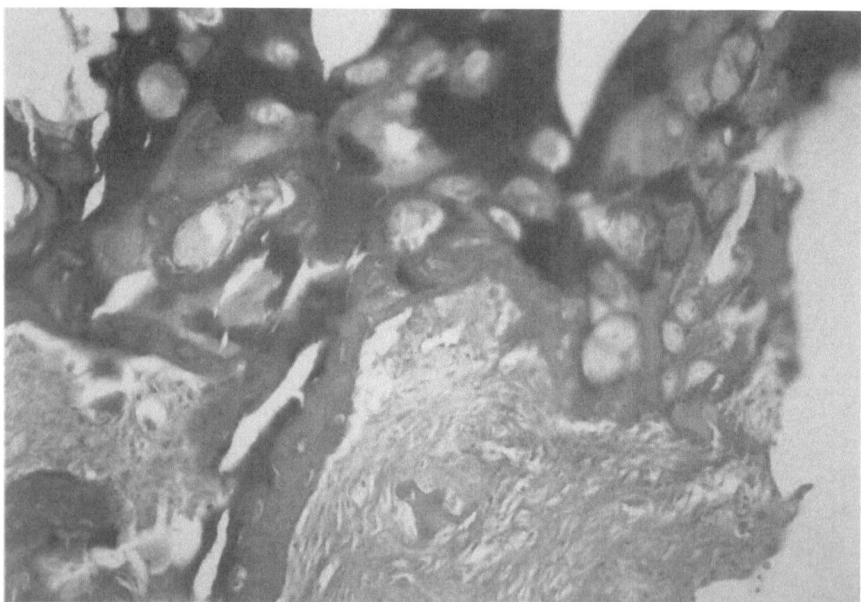

Fig. 4. Histological aspect of the condrodystrophic area, showing the presence of cartilage at a stage of maturation not compatible with the age of the patient, as well as pyrosis which upset the bony trabeculae

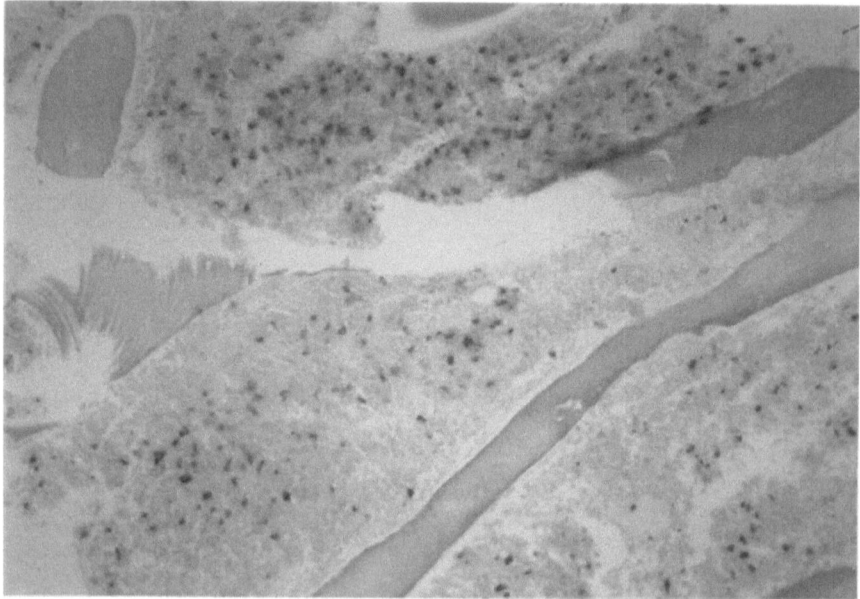

Fig. 5. Histological aspect using Perl, test for iron shows the presence of macrophages containing iron; this pigment is evident even outside, and the deposit is therefore ubiquitous

The histological finding concerning the condrodystrophic area, which are not dependent on the age of the patient, shows the cartilage at different stages of maturation, with fibrosis toward the medullar front (Fig. 4). In the calcification front section, fibrosis penetrates the trabecular bone. Using Perl's method, it becomes evident that iron is ubiquitous in pathological tissue (Fig. 5).

The EDAX technique showed that iron corresponded to 2.26 % of the weight of the sample. The presence of zinc and copper was also reported.

Discussion

Present therapeutic protocols have modified the clinical picture of thalassemic transfusion-dependent patients. Typical radiographic aspects [9] such as the "hair-on-end" appearance, the enlarged diaphyseal channel, and the reduction of cortical thickness have practically disappeared; the picture of osteoporosis is diminished [10], and the cartilaginous lesions have changed. In particular, cartilaginous lesions are typical of growth age [1], and they are easily found, therefore, in thalassemic patients who have been subjected, since their first months of life, to the modern therapeutic protocols characterized by a hypertransfusion regimen and the subsequent iron-chelation therapy. In older patients, who have received a less intense transfusion regimen and less intense iron-chelation therapy, the damage to the metaphyseal cartilage is indirectly documented by dysmetria [11] and deviation of the axes of the limbs [2]. The new generation of thalassemic subjects must face new and characteristic metaphyseal lesions [5–8]. These cartilaginous alterations show important morphological differences compared with the lesions observed and described in the past by various authors [9, 12, 13]. The radiological, ultrastructural, and chemical studies we carried out on our thalassemic patients show lesions of the examined structures. Moreover, radiographic surveys show a characteristic sclerotic wall of variable thickness, whose morphological characteristics are similar to those in other forms of condrodystrophy such as scurvy and rickets. In particular, computerized tomography and magnetic resonance imaging reveal a strucutral alteration of the metaphyseal interface which turns toward the front of calcification. The tissue is rich in cells that invade the trabecular bone structure.

The presence of a condrodystrophic picture in spite of continous therapeutic improvements shows that the cartilage is among the tissues most involved in thalassemia major. The clear involvement of the developing cartilage seems to show that the alteration of the Ca-P balance, due to endocrine and/or enzyme metabolic factors, is an important pathogenetic cause [14, 15]. Total body skeletal Tc99m scintigraphy shows that condrodystrophic areas appear hypointerceptive compared with other areas like the tibia and the proximal femur. Such a result ist the expression of a slowed calcium turnover. We do not deal here with the pathogenetic interpretation of these cartilaginous lesions. According to some authors, both an excessive dosage of desferrioxamine and iron-chelation therapy administered too early can play a pathogenetic role [5–8]. In some clinical cases, the decrease of the dosage induced a clinical improvement of the lesion. We think it important to report that we never administered desferrioxamine doses higher than 50 mg/kg body wt. per day, while subcutaneous iron-chelation therapy was started in almost all cases after 3 years of age. Moreover, the reduction of desferrioxamine from 50 to 25 mg/kg body wt. per day did not cause, after a year, any clear change in the evolution of the lesion. These results made us less optimistic regarding the prognosis of these lesions, which in their severest forms lead to deviation and dysmetria of the limbs [11]. Therefore, pathogenetic causes should be further investigated in order to find preventive measures and/or therapy to treat thalassemic condrodystrophy.

References

1. Giuzio E, Bria M, Brancati C (1991) Le alterazioni scheletriche nella thalassemia major. GIOT 17: 277–283
2. Colavita M, Orazi C, Danza SM, Falappa P, Fabbri R (1987) Premature epiphyseal fusion and extramedullary hematopoiesis in thalassemia. Skeletal Radio 16: 533–538
3. Currarino G, Erlandom M (1964) Premature fusion of epiphysis in Cooley anemia. Bone Joint Surg 83: 656–664
4. Esposito L, Ferrara M, Furante A (1976) Rilievi sull'accrescimento staturale e sulle maturazione scheletrica sulla talassemia mayor in rapporto alla terapia emotrasfusiva. Pediatria 84: 235–246
5. Podda G, Fodde M, Pirastu GF (1987) Preliminari considerazioni sulle alterazioni scheletriche in pazienti affetti da talassemia major trattati con deferoxamina. Atti 3rd SIRMN, Cagliari, pp 311–315
6. Brill PW, Winchester P, Giardina PJ (1991) Deferoxamine – induced bone dysplasia in patients with thalassemia major. A JR 156: 561–565
7. Orzincolo C, Scutellari P, Castaldi G (1992) Growth plate injury of the long bones in treated β-thalassemia. Skeletal Radiol 21: 39–44
8. De Virgillis S, Congia M, Frau F (1989) Deferoxamine-induced growth retardation in patients with thalassemia major. J Pediatr 113: 661
9. Model B, Berdoukas V (1984) The clinical approach to thalassaemia. Grune and Stratton New York
10. Giuzio E, Bria M, Bisconte MG, Brancati C L'Osteopenia nei thalassemici politrasfusi. Nostra esperienza. Chir Organi Mov 76: 369–374
11. Giuzio E, Bria M, Misasi M, Brancati L (1991) Le dismetrie degli arti inferiori nella thalassemia major. GIOT [suppl] 129–132
12. Middlemiss GM, Raper A (1966) Skeletal changes in the haemoglobinopathies. J Bone Joint Surg [Br] 48: 693–702
13. Radici M, Galloni O (1977) Le alterazioni scheletriche nella malattia di Cooley. Arch Osp S Anna 20: 885–889
14. Ramazzina E, Nardi A, Luisetto G, Chiavilli F (1986) Metabolismo minerale e scheletrico nella beta talassemia. Atti Accad Sci Ferrara 63: [Suppl] 251–263
15. Puxeddu L, Floris G, Murras MC (1984) II metabolismo calcico nell'osteopatia talassemica. Ortop Traumatol Oggi 4

Glucose Intolerance and Diabetes in Thalassaemia major

B. Wonke and J. I. Hanslip

The management of homozygous β-thalassaemia involves regular blood transfusions and subcutaneous infusions of the iron-chelating agent desferrioxamine (DFX) [1]. This optimal treatment appears to ensure good health in the long term, if DFX chelation begins in early childhood and is complied with, and if there is no evidence of viral hepatitis, then the patients can be expected to survive for an indefinite duration. Most of the complications of thalassaemia major are attributable to transfusion-transmitted viruses causing liver disease and to iron overload. The latter may be the result of economic circumstance, late onset of iron-chelation therapy or poor compliance with DFX treatment. In iron overload the excess iron which is deposited in the tissues causes damage. The mechanisms by which iron damages the organs have only recently been identified [2]. Toxicity begins when the iron load in a particular tissue exceeds the tissue or blood binding capacity of iron, and large quantities of free nontransferrin iron appear. This "free iron" is a catalyst of the production of oxygen species that damage cells and peroxidize membrane lipids, leading to cell destruction. The liver has a large capacity for producing proteins which bind the iron and store it in the form of ferritin and haemosiderin. However, eventually cirrhosis develops, which may be accelerated by chronic hepatits B or C viruses. In the pancreas iron deposition in the interstitial cells results in excessive collagen deposition and defective microcirculation. Impaired oxygen supply eventually leads to insulin deficiency [3]. This greatly contributes to the multifactorial pathology of the development of glucose intolerance and diabetes in thalassaemia major (Fig. 1).

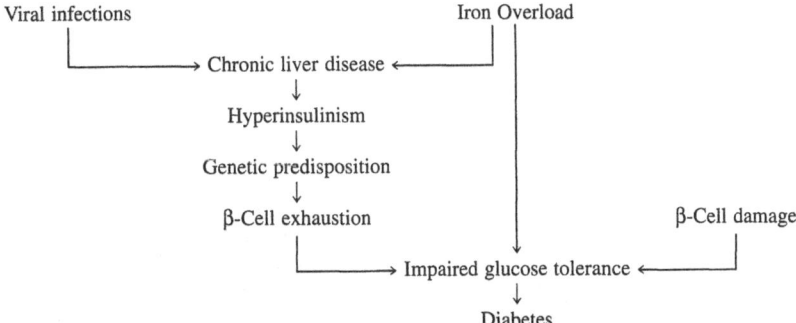

Fig. 1. Pathogenetics of glucose intolerance and diabetes in thalassaemia major

S. Andò et al. (Eds.)
Endocrine Disorders in Thalassemia
© Springer-Verlag Berlin Heidelberg 1995

Table 1. Incidence of IGT in thalassaemia major in the Mediterranean

No. of patients	Age range (mean years)	IGT no. (%)	Observations	Reference
19	(15.1)	11 (57.8)	Serum ferritin, AST and ALT as in controls	E. Tutor et al. (1992) Turkey
191	12–29	41 (21.4)	Serum ferritin > than controls	M. Karagiorga et al. (1992) Greece
90	10–29	21 (23.3)	Hypogonadism 9% Hypothyroidism 40% Hypoparathyroidism 12%	S. Anastasi et al. (1992) Italy

Table 2. Incidence of diabetes in thalassaemia major in the Mediterranean

No. of patients	Age range (mean years)	IGT no. (%)	Observations	Reference
150	13–25 (17.5)	10 (6.6)	Ferritin > 5000 ng/ml	S. Grutta et et al. (1992) Italy
191	12–29	9 (4.7)	Ferritin > than controls	M. Karagiorga et al. (1992) Greece
19	(15.1)	2 (10.5)	Serum ferritin, AST, ALT as in controls	E. Turor et al. (1992) Turkey

Table 3. Incidence of IGT and DM in thalassaemia major in the United Kingdom

No. of patients 72	Normal 31 (43%)	IGT 24 (33%)	DM 17 (24%)
Mean age at onset	23 years	22 years	20 years
Duration		1–2 years	
Mean number of transfusion	452	432	423
Mean serum ferritin (ng/ml)	2000	2500	5800

[a] Serum ferritin levels were significantly higher in IGT than in DM ($p = 0.0097$) and in DM than in controls ($p = 0.0035$).

The incidence of impaired glucose tolerance (IGT) in thalassaemia major varies between 11 and 24% (Table 1), that of diabetes mellitus (DM) between 2 and 10% (Table 2) in the Mediterranean countries; in the United Kingdom the incidences are 33% and 24% respectively (Table 3).

The onset of DM in the majority of patients is in the late teens, and both sexes are affected equally. IGT can present as early as at 10 years of age and it frequently precedes frank diabetes. IGT is asymptomatic, whilst DM itself presents with the classical symptoms, accompanied by ketosis or ketoacidosis [4]. At Whittington Hospital we have studied the incidence of IGT and DM, the age at presentation, the role of iron overload and genetic factors in thalassaemic patients. We have also studied the effect of intensive iron chelation in iron overloaded thalassaemia major patients and the role of a diabetic diet in preventing the development of DM in patients with IGT. Seventy-two patients (40 male, 32 female) aged between 6 and 43 years and receiving optimal treatment for thalassaemia were studied. Between 1977 and 1992, oral glucose tolerance tests (OGTT) were performed. Twenty-one patients had a single test and 34 two to five tests. Serum ferritin levels were estimated every 6 months, and transfusion history was assessed by multiplying the number of transfusion years by the average number of units transfused per year. All patients were questioned about family history of diabetes. The results (Table 3) clearly show that patients with high ferritin levels have an increased risk of developing DM. Genetic factors may also play an important role, as three patients who had a very strong family history of diabetes developed DM before the age of 17 years, despite very low serum ferritin levels. Biochemical diabetes may be reversible. Five patients with IGT who adhered to a strict diabetic diet and intensified iron chelation therapy for at least 1 year reverted to normal glucose metabolism on repeat testing. Good compliance with iron chelation is necessary to minimise the risk of DM. In patients with a strong family history of diabetes, IGT may present at an early age despite good compliance to DFX treatment and low serum ferritin levels. In this group yearly OGTT is recommended from the age of 10 years. In those with no family history of diabetes, good compliance to DFX treatment is necessary and yearly OGTT should be performed. A certain degree of islet cell function may be reversible, and thalassaemia major patients with IGT should be given advice on a diabetic diet and weight control with intensive iron chelation. The role of oral hypoglycaemic agents in IGT remains to be determined, as does that of alpha-interferon treatment in patients with viral induced chronic active hepatitis. Insulin requirements in thalassaemia patients with DM are variable and good control may be difficult to achieve. Long-term complications of diabetes should be looked for, in particular opthalmic and renal.

References

1. Cao A, Gabutti V, Masera G et al. (1992) Management protocol for the treatment of thalassemia patients. Handbook distributed by Thalassemia International Federation Cooley's Anemia Foundation, New York
2. Shinar E, Rachmitivitz EA (1990) Oxydative denaturation of red cells in thalassaemia. Semin haematol 27: 70–82
3. Iancu TC (1990) Biological and ultrastructural aspects of iron overload: an overview. Hemisphere, New York, pp 281–295
4. Davies SC, Wonke B (1991) The management of haemoglobinopathies. Baillieres Clin Haematol 4: 361–389

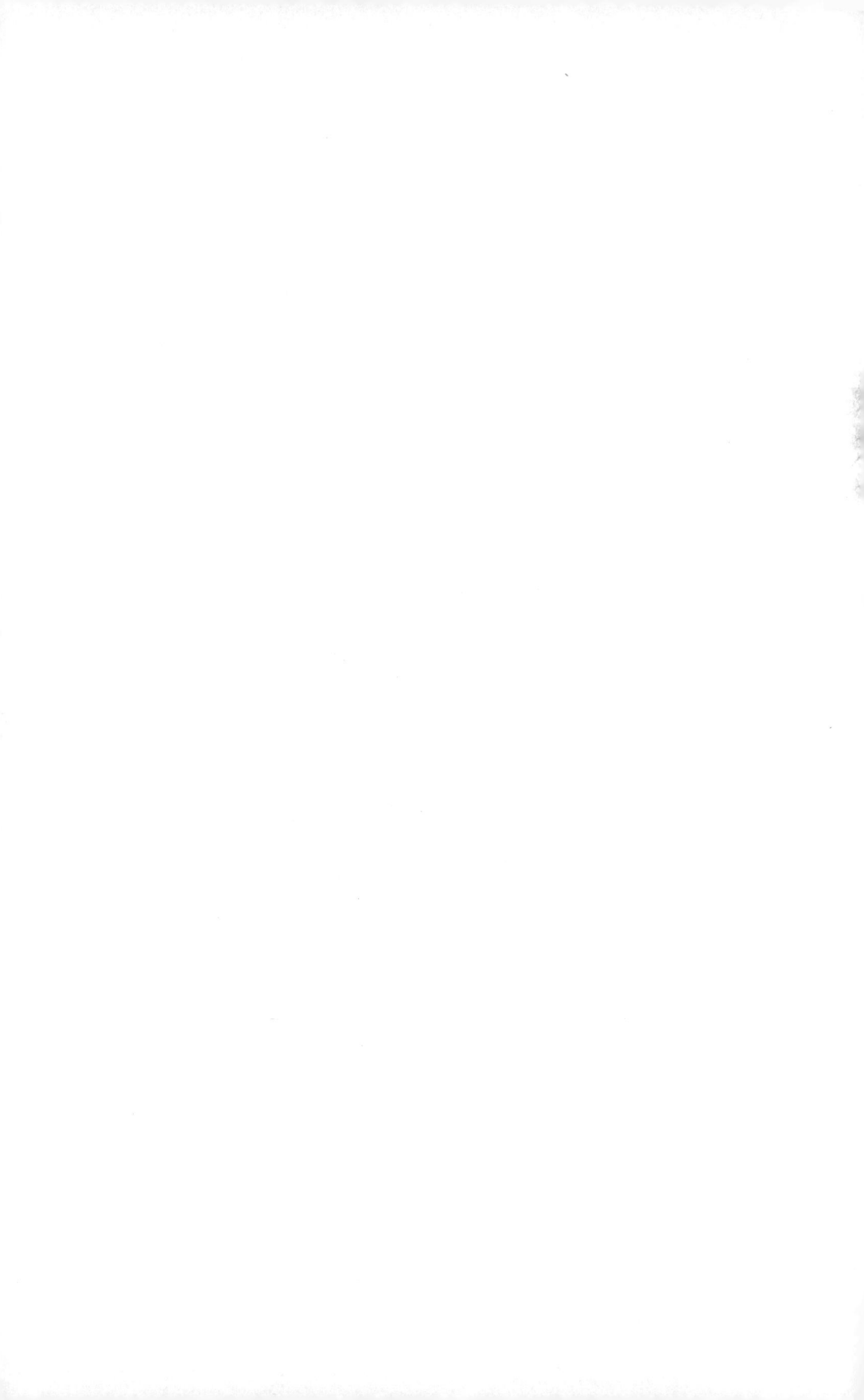

Pancreatic beta-Cell Function Before and After Bone Marrow Transplantation for Thalassemia

M. Galimberti, V. De Sanctis, G. Lucarelli, P. Polchi,
E. Angelucci, D. Baronciani, C. Giardini, B. Erer, J. Gaziev,
R. Balducci, and C. Vullo

Diabetes mellitus and impaired glucose tolerance are complications of thalassemic major patients treated by hypertransfusion schemes and chelation therapy. Diabetes in thalassemic patients seems to be the consequence of several factors. The iron overload damages the islet cells and also seems to decrease the sensitivity to insulin, which is compensated by increased secretion of insulin. So the diabetes may be due to a combination of insulin deficiency and insulin resistance. The insulin deficiency may be caused by either exhaustion of beta cells or beta-cell damage due to iron deposition, or a combination of these factors.

Another important factor is liver damage due to iron overload and viral infections [1–3]; the combination of these factors could explain the development of impaired glucose tolerance and, in time, insulin-dependent diabetes in thalassemia patients. This study was undertaken to evaluate the impact of bone marrow transplation on beta-pancreas function in thalassemic patients.

Materials and Methods

This study enrolled 93 patients without clinical signs of diabetes who had undergone bone marrow transplantation (BMT) at our center at least 2 years before our evaluation. The mean age was 11 years (range 3–16 years) pretransplant; 12 patients were in class 1, 53 in class 2, and 23 in class 3; five were unclassifiable [4]. All patients were prepared for transplantation with busulphan (BU) 14 mg/kg and cyclophosphamide (CY) 200 mg/kg and received cyclosporin (CSA) and steroids as GVHD prophylaxis [5, 6].

Oral glucose tolerance tests (OGTT) and tests of insulin response (IR) were performed after administration of 1.75 g glucose per kilogram body wt. up to a maximum of 100 g, and blood samples were obtained at 0, 30, 60, 90, 120, and 180 min for measurement of serum glucose and insulin.

The values of serum glucose were compared with the levels considered normal by the National Diabetes Data Group [7], while the serum levels of insulin were compared with those found in a group of normal children in the same age-group.

S. Andò et al. (Eds.)
Endocrine Disorders in Thalassemia
© Springer-Verlag Berlin Heidelberg 1995

Results and Discussion

Before transplantation several types of glucose disturbance were found in this group of patients. The responses to the OGTT were divided into three types: normal, impaired, and diabetic, the results of IR in four: normal, increased, delayed, and decreased. In Tabel 1 the results of OGGT and IR pretransplant are summarized. The pretransplant OGGT was normal in 55 % of the patients, impaired in 42 %, and diabetic in 3 %, while the IR was found to be normal in 52 patients, delayed in 30, decreased in five, and increased in six.

The percentage of thalassemic patients with an impaired OGTT is higher in our study than that described in other studies [8, 9], probably because our group of patients is heterogeneous with respect to the conventional treatment and also to the molecular basis of the disease.

We considered different parameters to evaluate their influence on glucose metabolism: the Pesaro risk class for transplant, age, transaminases, and the ferritin serum level. The transaminases were not significantly lower in the group of patients with normal OGTT, while age, ferritin level and risk class were found to be generally significant. These results are summarized in Table 2.

During the first several months after transplantation we observed an alteration of glucose metabolism in some patients. Of 51 patients with normal glucose metabolism pre-transplantation, six (11 %) had mild hyperglycemia that resolved simply by diet, while of the 40 patients with impaired metabolism, 12 (30%) had mild hyperglycemia, six (16%) required insulin treatment, two (6%) required glibenclamide treatment, and two (6%) developed insulin-dependent diabetes. The patients who received insulin and glibenclamide treatment had acute GVHD and needed steroids to cure it. The patients received diabetic treatment for 1–16 months and then stopped both treatment and diet. The two patients who developed insulin-dependent diabetes had liver cirrhosis before and after transplantation and one had a diabetic brother.

Between 1 and 7 years after the transplantation we reevaluated glucose tolerance in 55 of the 93 patients in this study and found a significant statistical improvement.

Table 1. Oral glucose tolerance and insulin response Pretransplant

	Insulin Response			
Oral glucose tolerance	Normal	Increased	Delayed	Decreased
Normal ($n = 51$)	43	1	6	1
Impaired ($n = 40$)	9	5	24	2
Diabetic ($n = 2$)	–	–	–	2

Table 2. Factors influencing pretransplant glucose tolerance

	Normal	Impaired	p
Class 1 (n)	11	1	0.005
Class 2/3 (n)	36	38	
Age (years) average	10	12	0.003
ALT (mU/ml) avaverage	38	44	0.49
Ferritin (ng/ml) average	2210	3352	0.002

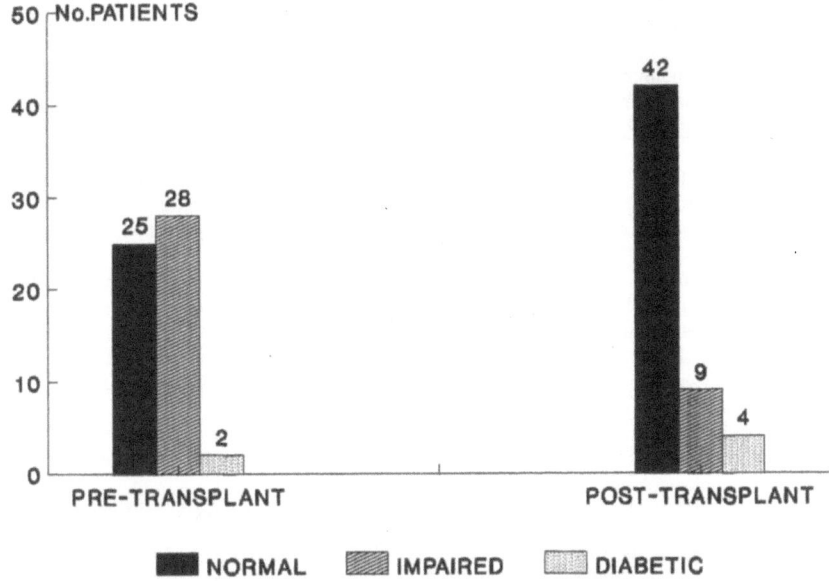

Fig. 1. Oral glucose tolerance before and after bone marrow transplantation

Of 25 patients with normal glucose metabolism prior to transplantation only one had an impaired metabolism post transplantation; this patient's liver biopsy worsened. Of 28 patients with impaired metabolism before transplantation, there after seven had impaired metabolism, two developed diabetes one with other endocrine alterations had a diabetic glucose intolerance, treated only with diet, and 18 showed an improvement of glucose metabolism with a normal OGTT. Of the two patients with a diabetic OGTT prior to transplantation, after the transplant one whose liver biopsy was improved thereafter had an impaired OGTT, while the other had insulin-dependent diabetes.

In Fig. 1 are summarized the OGTT results for these 55 patients before and after the transplantation. The improvement of OGTT seen after transplantation is statistically significant ($p = 0.002$).

Four patients who had an improvement of glucose metabolism required hormone treatment to help their pubertal development After 6–12 months of hormone therapy these patients had normal serum glucose values but impaired glucose metabolism, so we treated them by diet.

This study demonstrates that the conditioning regimen for transplantation with BU and CY and CSA used for GVHD prophylaxis does not affect the pancreatic beta-cell function. In some patients who were treated with steroids we observed an alteration of glucose metabolism that resolved in a few months. Only three patients with impaired OGTT prior to transplantation and with liver cirrhosis showed a worsening of pancreatic beta-cell function. The iron overload and the liver damage before transplantation are important factors for the outcome of glucose metabolism thereafter. In our study, 18 patients showed an improvement of glucose metabolism once they became ex-thalassemic after transplantation.

References

1. Merkel PA, Simonson DC, Amiel SA et al. (1988) Insulin resistance and hyperinsulinemia in patients with thalassemia major treated by hypertransfusion. N Engl J Med 318: 809–814
2. Vullo C, De Sanctis V, Katz M et al. (1990) Endocrine abnormalities in thalassemia. NY Acad Sci 612: 293–310
3. De Sanctis V, D'Ascola G, Wonke B (1986) The development of diabetes mellitus and chronic liver disease in long-term chelated beta-thalassaemia patients. Postgrad Med J 62: 831–836
4. Lucarelli G, Galimberti M, Polchi P et al. (1990) Bone marrow transplantation in patients with thalassemia. N Engl J Med 322: 417–421
5. Lucarelli G, Polchi P, Galimberti M et al. (1985) Marrow transplantation for thalassemia following busulphan and cyclophosphamide. Lancet 1: 1355–1357
6. Lucarelli G, Galimbert M, Polchi P et al. (1987) Marrow transplantation in patients with advanced thalassemia. N Engl J Med 316: 1050–1055
7. National Diabetes Data Group (1979) Classification and diagnosis of diabetes mellitus and other categories of glucose intolerance. Diabetes 28: 1039–1057
8. Ladis V, Theodorides C, Athanassaki C et al. (1991) Disturbance and management of glucose metabolism in thalassemic patients (Abstr.). 4th International Conference of Thalassemia and the Hemoglobinopathies, Nice, 231
9. De Sanctis V, Zurlo MG, Senesi E et al. (1988) Insulin-dependent diabetes in thalassaemia. Arch Dis Child 63: 58–62

A Multicenter Study on Endocrine Disorders in Thalassemia – Introduction*

V. de Sanctis, with S. Andò and C. Pintor

The distribution of β-thalassemia major throught out the world has clearly shown the highest prevalence along a belt which includes the Mediterranean area and spans through the Middle East, to India and East Asia. In 1988 the WHO reported that 240,000 children per year are born with a major hemoglobinopathy – 20% with thalassemias and 80% with the sickle cell syndrome. The total number of thalassemic patients transfused and followed up at Italian centers estimated on December 31, 1984 was 4497.

During the past 20 years endocrine complications in thalassemia have been an area of tremendous interest to clinicians and scientists working in many different fields. Expansion and subspecialization in endocrinological investigations indicate an ongoing, healthy developmental process; neverthless, they carry the risk of fragmenting the single body into uncollated segments and mark the current approach to endocrine complications in thalassemia as too sophisticated.

For this reason, I am certain that all of us are grateful to the organizing comittee for having planned this International Mediterranean Conference and for giving us an opportunity to collect and share the experiences from different countries.

Prof. Andò has asked me to introduce a round table, based on my personal experience with the multicenter study that we have organized in the past 3 years in Italy on endocrine complications in thalassemia. We met for the first time in March 1989 at the Pediatric Endocrine Meeting in Pisa, and our primary aims were to obtain more information on the incidence of endocrine complications in thalassemia, to plan future studies, and do an in-depth analysis of the data obtained. A standard form was specially designed to record all the information that we required. At present we are using a particular form for each endocrine complication.

I believe that our study is useful for many reasons:

1. To get to know each other, to compare experiences and to plan for the future.
2. To obtain more information on the incidence of endocrine complications in thalassemia, as data in the literature concern only small groups of patients.
3. To elucidate the problems that must be dealt with in the near future.
4. To standardize the criteria for a diagnosis of endocrine dysfunction. As a result of this the diagnoses of arrest of puberty, hypoparathyroidism, and different types of hypothyroidism are now more accurate than in the past.

---

* This is an introduction to the following three chapters.

S. Andò et al. (Eds.)
Endocrine Disorders in Thalassemia
© Springer-Verlag Berlin Heidelberg 1995

In addition, it is useful for colleagues working in small hospitals and following only a few patients to obtain a broader view. They were enthusiastic about participating in this survey and being actively being in the study.

During our study we have also learned that some problems are only partially studied and treated, and for this reason a few months ago we started a multicenter study on short stature and growth hormone deficiency in thalassemia. I hope that I have given you a rough idea of how interesting and helpful this study has been for us. We would be very pleased to support the extension of this study in other countries with advice based on the knowledge we have gained, and we would also be prepared to participate actively.

Endocrine Pathology in Thalassemia

D. Sonakul

Introduction

Patients with thalassemia suffer from anemia, accelerated intramedullary and extra-medullary erythropoiesis, and iron overload due to hemolysis and increased absorption from the gastrointestinal tract, with deleterious effects on internal organs and tissues [2, 7–9]. With modern treatment and longer survival, endocrine dysfunction assumes greater importance [1, 3–5]. This study was carried out in an attempt to correlate such dysfunction with pathologic findings in major endocrine organs.

Materials and Methods

Autopsy protocols and histologic sections of 81 thalassemic patients in this study were taken from the files of the Pathology Department, Siriraj Hospital, from the period 1972–1990. The material consisted of eight cases of beta-thalassemia major (beta-thal), 60 cases of beta-thalassemia with hemoglobin E disease (beta-thal/HbE), and 13 cases of hemoglobin H disease (HbH), the patients ranging in age from 6 months to 67 years; 72 of the patients were less than 25 years old and seven of the eight beta-thal patients died in their first or second decade. Four of the eight beta-thal patients, 38 of the 60 beta-thal/HbE patients, and six of the 13 HbH patients were male. The spleen had been removed 2–20 years previously from six beta-thal, 49 beta-thal/HbE, and two HbH patients. All had received minimal blood transfusion. Histologic sections were formalin fixed, paraffin embedded, and stained with hematoxylin and eosin (H&E), Gomori's iron stain (Fe), and Masson's trichrome and periodic acid-Schiff (PAS) stains where appropriate.

Results

Pituitary Gland

Sections of 17 pituitary glands were available, from three beta-thal and 14 beta-thal/HbE patients. Iron deposition was significant in only 19% of these pituitary glands, predominantly in older splenectomized patients, although a 19-year-old girl with beta-thal also had heavy iron deposition. Iron, when present, was found in the

S. Andò et al. (Eds.)
Endocrine Disorders in Thalassemia
© Springer-Verlag Berlin Heidelberg 1995

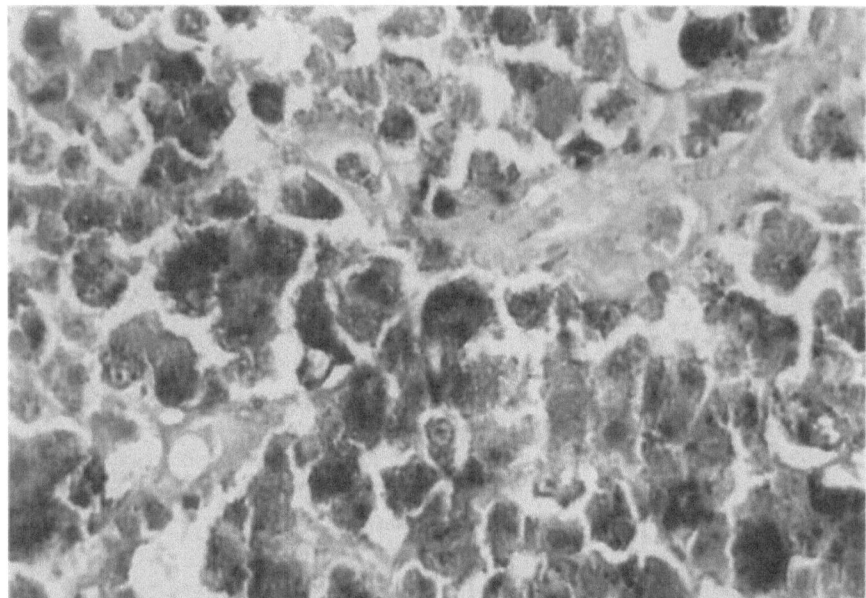

a

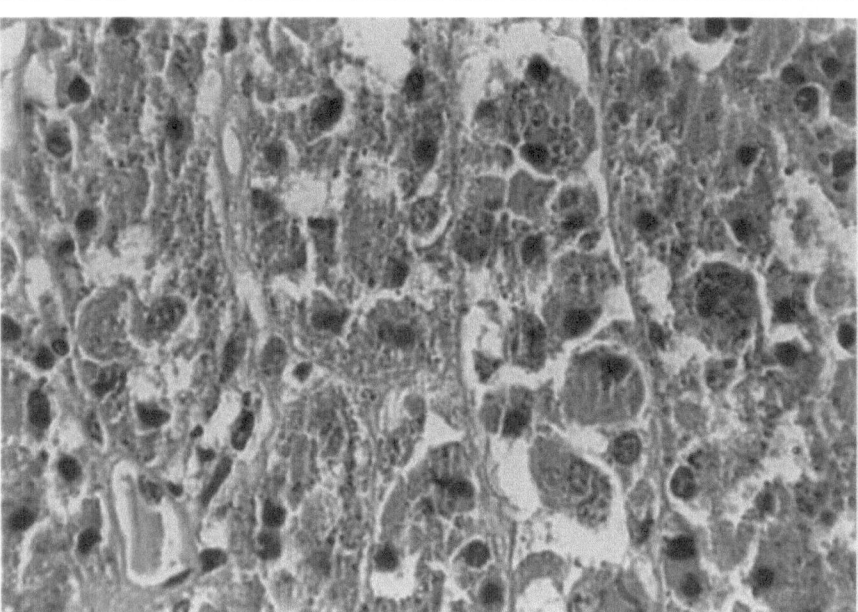

b

Fig. 1a, b. Pituitary gland: 32-year-old splenectomized man with beta-thal/HbE. **a** Moderate iron deposition. Fe, original magnification × 450; **b** extensive lipofuscin deposition. H & E, original magnification × 450

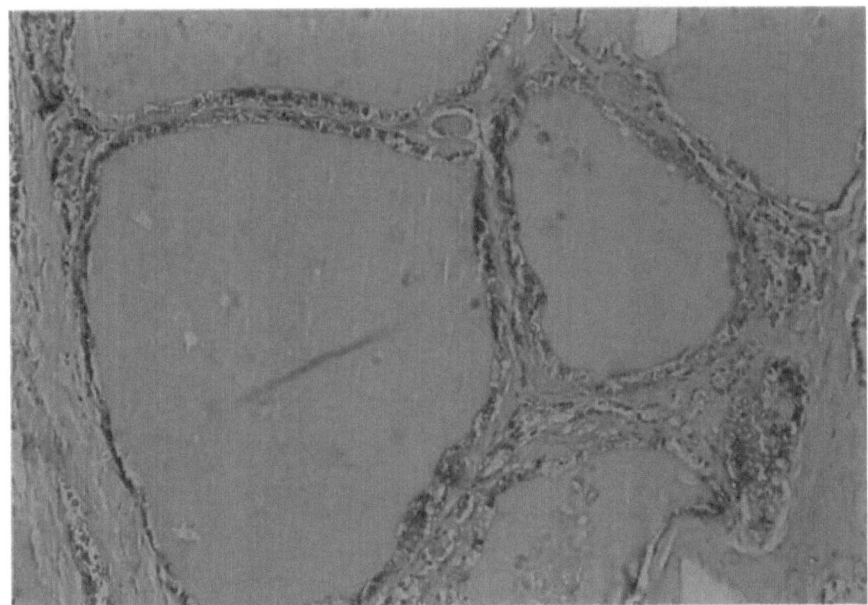

Fig. 2. Thyroid gland: 25-year-old splenectomized woman with beta-thal/HbE. Moderate siderosis with focal fibrosis. Fe, original magnification × 100

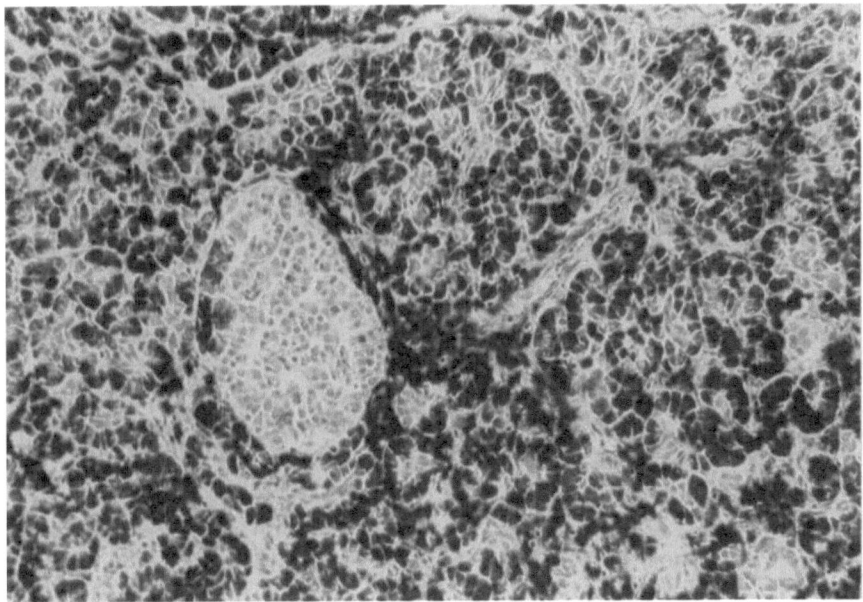

Fig. 3. Pancreas: 13-year-old splenectomized girl with beta-thal. Heavy siderosis in acinar cells, minimal in islet cells. Fe, original magnification × 100

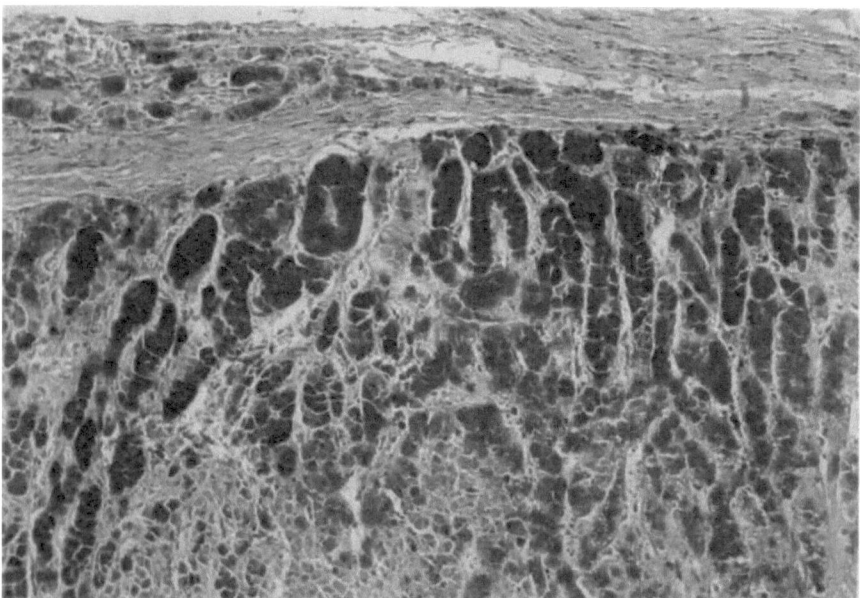

Fig. 4. Adrenal gland: 48-year-old splenectomized man with beta-thal/HbE. Heavy iron deposition in the zona glomerulosa with irregular extension into the zona fasciculata. Fe, original magnification × 100

anterior lobe, predominantly in acidophils and chromophobes or degranulated chromophils (Fig. 1a); none was found in the posterior lobe. Lipofuscin was found in virtually all cases, in all types of cells, sometimes to such a degree that the cells appeared ballooned (Fig. 1b). Fibrosis was minimal.

Thyroid Gland

Significant iron was found in seven of 24 thyroid glands available for study, with the heaviest deposition in thyroid glands from two beta-thal patients – a 9-year-old boy and a 24-year-old woman, accompanied by extensive fibrosis; three beta-thal/HbE patients had moderate iron deposition, and two others had extensive siderosis with slight focal fibrosis (Fig. 2). All these patients had been splenectomized. In some cases, follicular contents appeared blue tinged on iron stain. Two beta-thal/HbE patients had low to flat follicular epithelial cells, suggestive of hypofunction, and one had nodular goiter; no iron was seen in these three thyroid glands. Thyroid glands from two HbH patients appeared entirely normal.

Parathyroid Gland

Only six parathyroid glands were available for study, all from beta-thal/HbE patients. Two of these glands, from splenectomized patients aged 29 and 35 years,

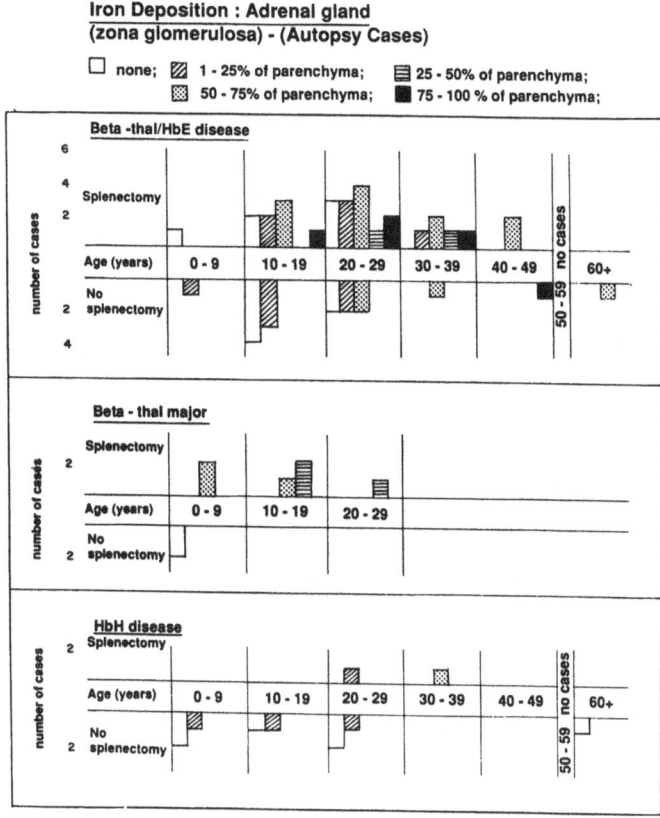

Fig. 5. Adrenal siderosis in splenectomized and nonsplenectomized patients in relation to age and type of thalassemia

showed moderate to heavy iron deposition; the remaining four showed minimal iron. Lipofuscin was seen in all six parathyroids, so much in some cases that the cells appeared ballooned. Fibrosis was not evident.

Pancreatic Islets

Iron deposition in pancreatic islets was slight in all three types of patients, including two who died in diabetic ketosis, while three nondiabetic patients as well as one diabetic had heavy iron deposition accompanied by fibrosis. Iron deposition increased with age and was heavier in splenectomized patients. Among the three types of thalassemia, iron deposition appeared at an earlier age and in greater quantity in patients with beta-thal, least in patients with HbH. The small amount of iron in the islets contrasted strongly with heavy deposition in the acini (Fig. 3); this was often accompanied by fibrosis, especially in older patients. Islets often appeared smaller if acinar and interstitial fibrosis was extensive. Lipofuscin was seen in islet cells from the age of 10 years and was often extensive, similar to lipofuscin deposition in the pituitary.

Adrenal Gland

Iron deposition was present in 35% of adrenal glands, extensively in three patients: an 18-year-old splenectomized woman with beta-thal and two splenectomized beta-thal/HbE patients, 25 and 48 years old; this last patient had frank Addison's disease. Deposition was mainly in the outer layers, particularly the zona glomerulosa; with heavier siderosis there was irregular extension into the zona fasciculata (Fig. 4). Even in patients with nodular cortical hyperplasia, iron deposition was heaviest in the outer layers of the individual nodules. In cases of heavy iron deposition, fine hemosiderin granules were also seen in ganglion cells of the adrenal medulla, though no iron was found in the zona reticularis in any of the cases. Iron deposition increased with age and was heaviest in splenectomized patients. Among the three types of thalassemia, iron appeared at an earlier age and was heaviest in beta-thal patients, least in HbH patients (Fig. 5), similar to the picture in pancreatic islets. Lipofuscin appeared in all layers of cortical cells from the age of 10 years and was often extensive. Cortical cells with and without iron, with and without lipofuscin, often appeared atrophic. Fibrosis was minimal.

Reproductive Organs

Secondary sexual characteristics were described as underdeveloped in 75% of patients, with absent axillary and pubic hair, flat breasts, and childlike external genitalia.

Eleven *testes* and four *prostate glands* from patients with beta-thal/HbE were available for study: six testes had juvenile seminiferous tubules and no Leydig cells, consistent with hypofunction; two patients, 18 and 35 years old, had normal testes; the testes from three other patients, aged 21, 35, and 47 years, had atrophic seminiferous tubules with extensive fibrosis, suggestive of later testicular failure; in fact, the 47-year-old patient had fathered five children before loss of libido ensued. None showed iron deposition. Three of the four prostate glands were juvenile, with small glands with minimal branching; the fourth was within normal limits.

Nine *ovaries* were available, all from beta-thal/HbE patients: seven, from women 17–35 years of age, were small and undeveloped; an ovary from a 26-year-old nonsplenectomized woman appeared almost normal in size but was cystic; one from a 50-year-old nonsplenectomized woman had prominent stromal cells and a few corpora albicantia, suggestive of previous ovulation. No iron deposition was seen.

Ten *uteri* were available for study. The uteri from two beta-thal patients aged 18 and 24 years as well as five of eight uteri from patients with beta-thal/HbE were tiny and juvenile with flat endometrium. The uterus from the 26-year-old woman with cystic ovaries described above was postpartum. Two other beta-thal/HbE uteri were normal, including that of the 50-year-old woman with ovarian corpora albicantia.

Discussion

The amount of visible iron in the form of hemosiderin in different organs did not always correlate with the degree of dysfunction. The pituitary gland has been called the conductor of the endocrine orchestra, and pituitary hypofunction was at least partly responsible for hypofunction of most endocrine organs, in particular growth and sexual retardation [1], yet only 19% our cases had significant iron in the pituitary gland. Thyroid hypofunction was seen in patients with and without thyroid siderosis. Christenson et al. [4] regarded low parathormone levels as the cause of osteoporosis and osteomalacia, yet iron was seen in only two of six parathyroid glands in our series; besides, thin bony trabeculae are due to marrow expansion from accelerated erythropoiesis as well as to parathyroid dysfunction. In European and American series [8, 9], as well as in ours [7], pancreatic islets were found to contain far less iron than acinar cells, though few symptoms could be attributed to the latter. Two of our patients who fit the description of "bronzed diabetes" had virtually no islet siderosis, and pigmentation in the skin was actually increased melanin, probably secondary to pituitary and/or adrenal dysfunction, and not iron. The endocrine organ with the greatest amount of iron was the adrenal gland, heaviest in the zona glomerulosa, though Canale et al. [3] described mineralocorticoid levels as within normal limits; conversely, Andò et al. [1] reported low cortisol levels, but the zona fasciculata contained little iron. Perhaps greater damage is done by invisible iron, in particular ferritin, or by the ubiquitous lipofuscin, which should be controllable with increased vitamin E.

Addendum

At the request of the editors, it is noted here that, whereas patients over the age of 15 years in our series received minimal blood transfusion, younger patients were transfused on an irregular basis, usually when anemia became severe. Patients receiving multiple transfusions comprised four of six children with beta-thal and three of ten children with beta-thal/HbE. Significant iron deposition was found in two splenectomized beta-thal patients: an 8-year-old boy with moderate siderosis of the pancreatic islets and adrenal cortex, and a 9-year-old boy with moderately heavy deposition in the thyroid gland, small amounts in the pancreatic islets and adrenal cortex, and none in the pituitary. Another 8-year-old splenectomized boy with beta-thal and a 4-year-old nonsplenectomized boy with beta-thal/HbE had small amounts of iron in the pancreatic islets and adrenal cortex. In the group of children not receiving multiple transfusions, one of two beta-thal and two of seven beta-thal/HbE children had detectable iron in the pancreatic islets and adrenal cortex. However, it is difficult to determine whether earlier and heavier iron deposition was due to multiple transfusions or to more severe disease in children requiring multiple transfusions.

Acknowledgements The author would like to thank Mr. Chaiyuth Buawatana and Mr. Vicha Sookpatdhee for their invaluable help with the illustrations.

References

1. Andò S, Giachetto C, Bria M et al. (1987) Endocrine correlates of adrenal and testicular function with circulating ferritin plasma levels in adult thalassemic patients. Birth Defects 23: 459–468
2. Bhamarapravati N, Na-Nakorn S, Wasi P, Tuchinda S (1967) Pathology of abnormal hemoglobin diseases in Thailand. I. Pathology of beta-thalassemia/hemoglobin E disease. J Clin Pathol 46: 745–758
3. Canale VC, Steinherz P, New M, Erlandson M (1974) Endocrine functions in thalassemia major. Ann NY Acad Sci 282: 333–345
4. Christenson RA, Pootrakul P, Burnell JM et al. (1987) Patients with thalassemia develop osteoporosis, osteomalacia and hypoparathyroidism, all of which are corrected by transfusion. Birth Defects 23: 409–416
5. Costin G, Kogut MD, Hyman CB, Ortega JA (1979) Endocrine abnormalities in thalassemia major. J Dis Child 133: 497–502
6. Hyman CB, Landing B, Alfin-Slater R et al. (1974) dl-Alpha-tocopherol, iron and lipofuscin in thalassemia. Ann NY Acad Sci 232: 211–220
7. Sonakul D, Pacharee P, Thakerngpol K (1988) Pathologic findings in 76 autopsy cases of thalassemia. Birth Defects 23: 157–176
8. Whipple GH, Bradford WL (1936) Mediterranean disease–thalassemia (erythroblastic anemia of Cooley). J Pediatr 9: 279–311
9. Witzleben CL, Wyatt JP (1961) The effect of long survival on the pathology of thalassaemia major. J Pathol Bacteriol 82: 1–12

Endocrine Complications
in Cyprian Thalassemic Patients

N. SKORDIS

Endocrine disturbances are commonly found in thalassaemic patients who are regularly transfused and receive chelation therapy [1]. Iron overload from blood transfusions results in deposits in many organs including the endocrine glands, causing endocrine dysfunction. The incidence of endocrinopathies in thalassemics has been reported to be high by several investigators [2, 3]. The gland most sensitive to iron deposition is thought to be the pituitary, so that thalassemics often have delayed puberty and hypogonadism.

In Cyprus, an island with a population of 744,000, the number of thalassemia patients is remarkable due to the relatively high incidence of the thalassemia gene. Most of our patients, however, are adolescents and adults as there has been a significant decrease in new thalassemics due to our prevention program.

Among 585 thalassemics we have 12 patients who developed insulin-dependent diabetes mellitus (IDDM) after the age of 15 years. The frequency of hypoparathyroidism and hypothyroidism is also very low, so that in this report we will address the issues of growth failure and hypogonadism, which are more commonly observed.

Growth Failure

Short stature is frequently observed in children and adolescents with thalassemia and cannot always be explained by defective growth hormone (GH) secretion, as most of the studies have demonstrated normal GH response to provocative stimuli [4–6]. Several other factors such as genotype, anemia, and chelation therapy appear to contribute to this complication [7]. It has also been reported that GH-induced somatomedin generation is impaired [8] and the 24-h secretion of GH is decreased [1] in thalassemics.

Growth failure in our thalassemics has been found to be the most common endocrine complication. We have studied 433 thalassemics, most of whom have already achieved final height as shown in Table 1. Standing and sitting heigth were measured using the Harpender Stadiometer. The results are shown in Table 2. It is clear that sitting height is much more frequently affected than standing height. It is also of interest that male patients suffer more frequently from short stature compared with female patients (Table 3). In patients with both standing and sitting height below the 3rd percentile the Z score of sitting height was significantly more than that of standing height in all age-groups of both sexes (Figs. 1, 2).

S. Andò et al. (Eds.)
Endocrine Disorders in Thalassemia
© Springer-Verlag Berlin Heidelberg 1995

Table 1. Age distribution of 433 patients

Sex	Age (years)	Number
Male-Female	0–12	25
Male	12–14	22
Female	12–16	37
Male	14–18	49
Female	16–18	32
Female	over 18	129
Male	over 18	139

Table 2. Percentage of patients suffering short stature and hypogonadism

Age-group	Standing height	Sitting height	Hypogonadism
0–12 (M + F)	16	36	
12–24 (M)	36	68	
12–16 (F)	24	78	
14–18 (M)	59	80	38
16–18 (F)	47	79	27
> 18 (M)	44	78	32
> 18 (F)	19	56	33

Table 3. Percentage of 433 patients suffering short stature

	Standing height	Sitting height
Male	47	82
Female	20	65
Overall	35	72

Based on these findings, it is clear that short stature is an important complication in thalassemia. Male patients appear to suffer growth failure more frequently than female patients. It is also obvious that sitting height is much more frequently and severely affected.

Growth Hormone Secretion

Growth hormone secretion was studied using conventional provocative stimuli such as insulin-induced hypoglycemia, clonidine, and L-dopa. In addition, the response of GH to growth hormone-releasing hormone (GHRH) was investigated in some patients. A GHRH test was performed in the morning following an overnight fast, while the patients were awake and during bed rest. All patients received GHRH in an i.v. bolus of 1 µg/kg body wt. On separate occasions these patients were tested with other stimuli in order to assess their GH secretion to conventional provocation.

We have evaluated 12 patients (nine male and three female) aged 11–15 years with growth failure using the GHRH test. All had been regularly transfused from early infancy and received chelation therapy with desferrioxamine. Prepubertal patients ($n = 6$) had delayed bone age (mean: 12 years) compared with chronological age (mean: 14.3 years). All had normal thyroid function and none of them had IDDM

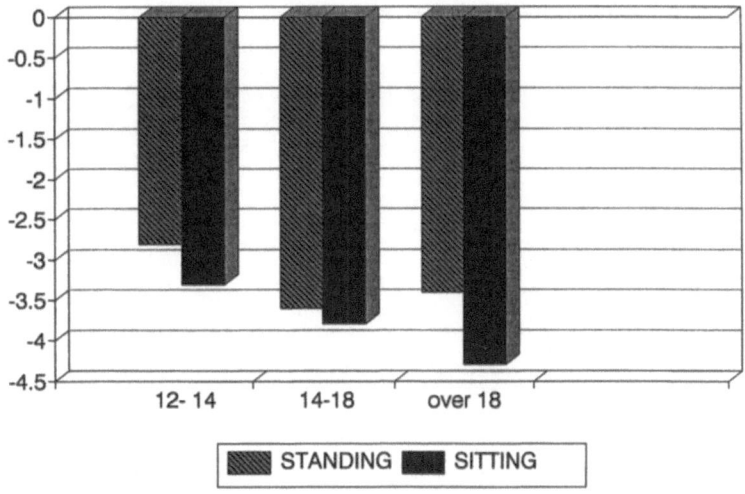

Fig. 1. Standard deviations in standing and sitting height in male age-groups

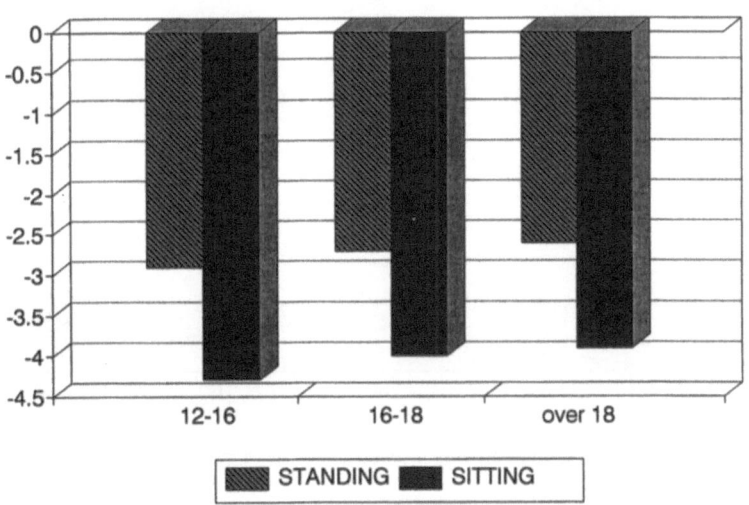

Fig. 2. Standard deviations in standing and sitting height in female age-groups

or impaired glucose tolerance. There was no evidence of chronic liver disease in any of these patients. In all patients GH secretion based on conventional provocative stimuli was found to be normal, as they all had values of GH more than 20 MIU/l. The mean ferritin level was 1955 ng/ml in the prepubertal patients and 1842 ng/ml in the pubertal ones.

Administration of GHRH evoked a rise of GH in all patients, shown in Fig. 3. The peak was found to occur 30 min following the injection in 50% of the patients,

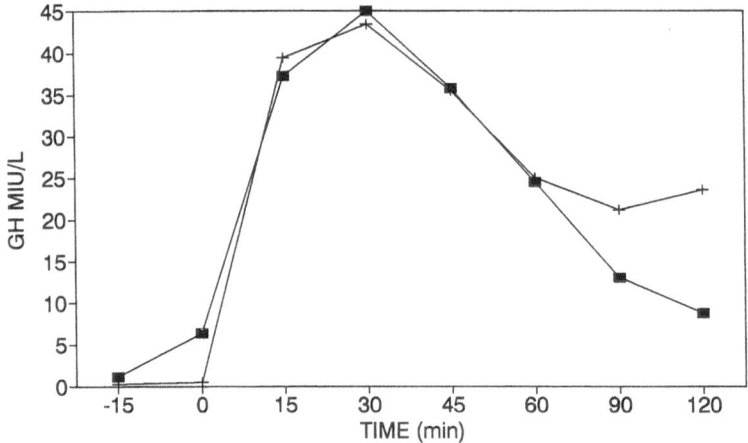

Fig. 3. Response of GH to GHRH in thalassemics (-■-, $n = 12$) and nonthalassemics (+, $n = 10$)

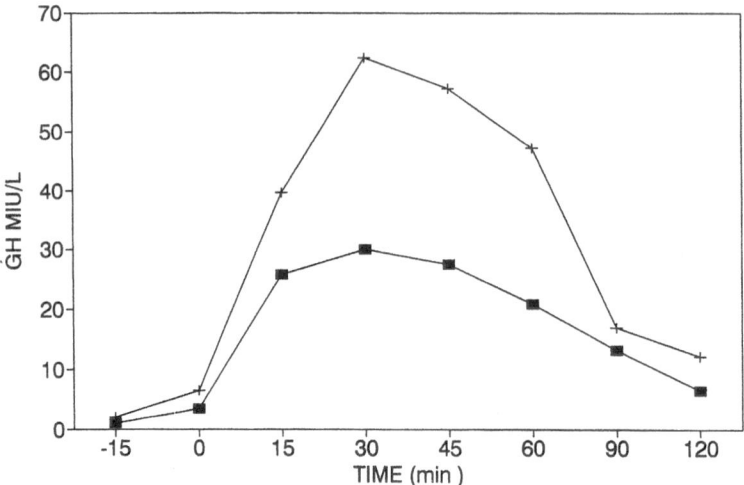

Fig. 4. Response of GH to GHRH in prepubertal (-■-, $n = 6$) and pubertal (+, $n = 6$) thalassemic patients.

whereas others demonstrated their peak values at 15 min, 45 min, or 60 min. It was also found that pubertal patients responded with a higher level of GH compared with prepubertal patients, as shown in Figs. 4 and 5.

Based on these findings from this relatively small number of patients, it seems that GH response to GHRH falls within the normal range. Prepubertal thalassemics demonstrate lower GH response compared with pubertal patients.

The early report by Pintor et al. [5] suggested impaired GH response to GHRH in thalassemia, which was not confirmed by subsequent studies [9]. It has been suggested that this discrepancy could be an age-related phenomenon, since the

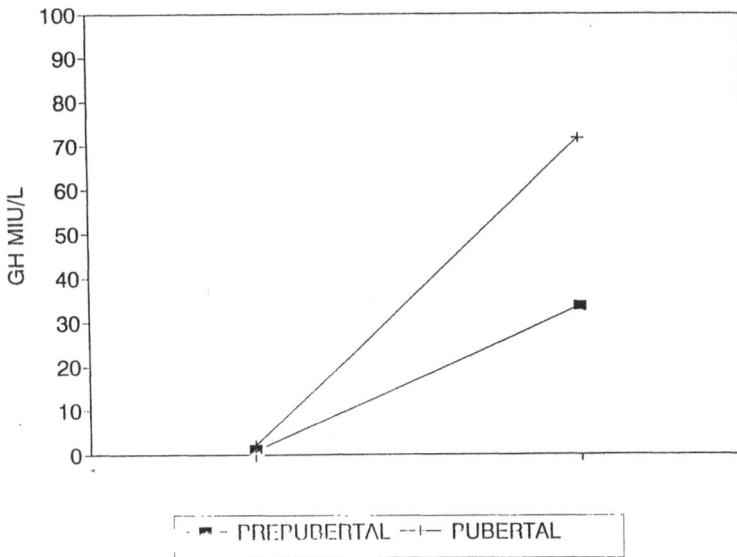

Fig. 5. Comparison of peak GH response to GHRH in prepubertal (-■-) and pubertal (+) patients

patients in the first study had a mean chronological age of 15.1 years, while in the second study the mean age was 7.6 years. From our results it appears that pubertal patients not only are able to preserve their pituitary function, but also respond with higher GH values compared with pre-pubertal patients.

Hypothalamic-Pituitary-Gonadal Axis in Male Thalassemics

Delayed, absent, or arrested pubertal development is a significant endocrinopathy in thalassemia [10]. Primary amenorrhea and secondary amenorrhea are frequently seen in female patients, while lack of sexual development and azoospermia are often found in male patients.

Although the etiology of hypogonadism in thalassemia has already been established by previous studies [11–13], this is the first report on the hypothalamic-pituitary-gonadal axis in thalassemics in Cyprus. The frequency of hypogonadism among our 433 examined thalassemics of different age-groups is shown in Table 2.

Hypogonadism in male thalassemics is manifested by delayed or arrested pubertal development, mostly as a result of gonadotropin deficiency and, in some instances, with additional testicular dysfunction.

We studied 51 male thalassemics aged 14–34 years, of whom 30 had delayed puberty or hypogonadism [mean testosterone (T): 1.8 nmol/l]: three were going through pubertal development (mean T: 9.2 nmol/l) and 18 were normal adults (mean T: 31.2 nmol/l). All received gonadotropin-releasing hormone (GnRH) at a dose of 100 µg as an i.v. bolus, and both FSH and LH were measured following stimulation for 2-h. Hypogonadal patients were additionally tested with Human Chorionic Gonadotropin (HCG) to evaluate testicular function.

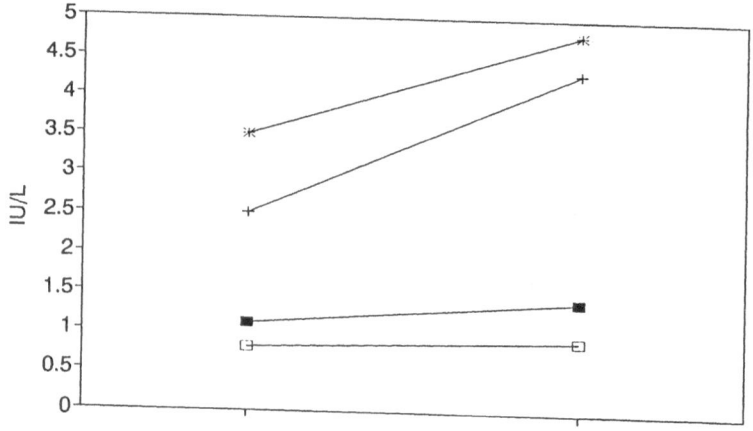

Fig. 6. Response of FSH to GnRH in 51 male thalassemics: ■, 30 patients with hypogonadism; +, three pubertal patients; *, 18 normal adult patients; □, five patients with multiple endocrinopathies

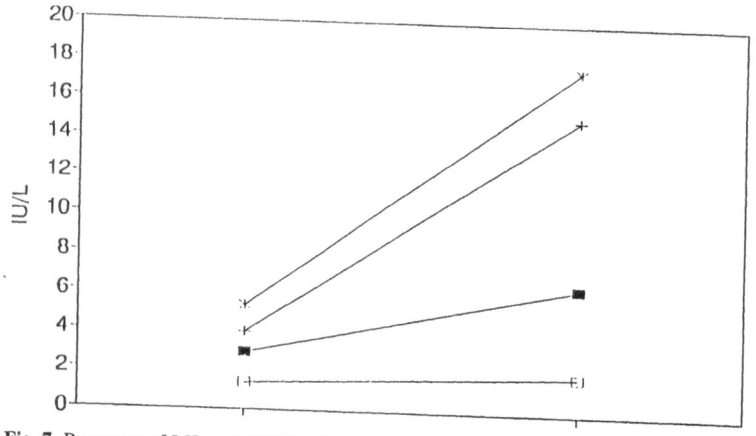

Fig. 7. Response of LH to GnRH in 51 male thalassemics: symbols as in Fig. 6

The response of FSH and LH in the different groups of patients is shown in Fig. 6 and Fig. 7, respectively. It is of interest that hypogonadal male patients with additional endocrinopathies demonstrated a complete absence of FSH and LH response compared with those who had no other endocrine disorder. The results of the HCG test revealed an excellent rise of the testosterone level from a baseline value of 1.8 nmol/l to a post-stimulation value of 23.4 nmol/l.

These results indicate that hypogonadism in male thalassemics is primarily a result of pituitary dysfunction, with the FSH response being almost absent. Hypogonadal patients with additional endocrinopathies show more severe damage, indicating more severe hemosiderosis. Normal testicular function was established in all our patients. Satisfactory pituitary response was shown in all normal adult male thalassemics.

References

1. Vullo C, De Sanctis V, Katz M et al. (1991) Endocrine abnormalities in thalassemia. Ann NY Acad Sci 445: 293–310
2. Canale V, Steinherz P, New M, Erlandson M (1974) Endocrine function in thalassemia major. Ann NY Acad Sci 232: 333–345
3. Flynn DM, Fairmen A, Jackson D, Clayton BE (1976). Hormonal changes in thalassemia major. Arch Dis Child 51: 828
4. Kuo B, Zaino E, Roginski MS (1968). Endocrine function in thalassemia major. J Clin Endocrinol Metab 28: 805–808
5. Pintor C, Cella SG, Manso P et al. (1986) Impaired growth hormone (GH) response to GH-releasing hormone in thalassemia major. J Clin Endocrinol Metab 62: 263–267
6. Scacchl M, Danesl L, De Martin M et al. (1991) Treatment with biosynthetic growth hormone of short thalassaemic patients with impaired growth hormone secretion. Clin Endocrionol (Oxf) 35: 335–338
7. Kattamis C, Liakopoulou T, Kattamis A (1990) Growth and development in children with thalassaemia major. Acta Paediatr Scand [Suppl] 366: 111–117
8. Pomarede R, Girot R, Constapt S et al. (1984) Effet du traitement hématologique sur la croissance et le développement pubertaire des enfants atteints de thalassémie majeure. Arch Fr Pediatr 41: 255–259
9. Leger J, Girot R, Crosnier H et al. (1989) Normal growth hormone (GH) response to GH-releasing hormone in children with thalassemia major before puberty: a possible age-related effect. Clin Endocrinol Metab 69: 453–456
10. Borgna-Pignatti C, De Stefano P, Zonta L et al. (1985) Growth and sexual maturation in thalassaemia major. J Pediatr 106: 150–155
11. Kletzky OA, Costin G, Marrs RP et al. (1979) Gonadotrophin insufficiency in patients with thalassaemia major. J Clin Endocrinol Metab 48: 901–905
12. De Sanctis V, Vullo C, Katz M (1988) Gonadal function in patients with b-thalassaemia major. J Clin Pathol 41: 133-137
13. De Sanctis V, Vullo C, Katz M (1988) Induction of spermatogenesis in thalassaemia. Fertil Steril 50: 969–975

Thalassemia and Endocrinopathies: Multicenter Study of 3092 Patients

ITALIAN WORKING GROUP ON ENDOCRINE COMPLICATIONS IN NON-ENDOCRINE DISEASES[*]

Introduction

Data regarding the prevalence of endocrine dysfunction in patients with β-thalassaemia major are limited [1, 2]. We report the results of a collaborative study of endocrine complications in a large series of patients with β-thalassemia major followed in pediatric and hematology departments throughout Italy.

Patients and Methods

The working group of the Italian Endocrine Pediatric Society (SIEDP) on endocrine complications in non-endocrine diseases started in March 1989 by sending a questionnaire to 29 centers treating a total of 1943 β^0 or β^+ thalassemia major patients, 46 % of

* *Steering committee:* V. De Sanctis, Department of Pediatrics, S. Anna Hospital, Ferrara; C. Pintor, Department of Pediatric Endocrinology, University of Cagliari, Cagliari.
Participants: M. Ughi, Department of Pediatrics, S. Anna Hospital, Ferrara; MC. Aliquò, Microcitemia Center, Rome; S. Anastasi, Microcitemia Center, Catania; S. Andò, Department of Cellular Biology, University of Calabria, Cosenza; C. Brancati, Microcitemia Center, Cosenza; M.A. Bruno, Microcitemia Center, Matera; G.A. Cambosu, Department of Pediatrics, Carbonia; A. Castiota Scanderbeg, Department of Pediatrics, University of Parma, Parma; F. Chiavilli, Blood Bank, Rovigo; C. Ciaccio, Microcitemia Center, Sciacca, Agrigento; C. Cianciulli, Microcitemia Center, S. Eugenio Hospital, University of Rome, Rome; M. Cisternino, Department of Pediatrics, University of Pavia, Pavia; G. D'Ascola, Microcitemia Center, Reggio Calabria; F. Di Gregorio, Department of Pediatrics, University of Catania, Catania; L. Esposito, Department of Pediatrics, Hematology Service, University of Naples, Naples; M.C. Galati, Microcitemia Center, A. Pugliese Hospital, Catanzaro; D. Gallisai, Microcitemia Center, Division of Therapy University of Sassari, Sassari; M.R. Gamberini, Department of Pediatrics, S. Anna Hospital, Ferrara; C. Gerardi, Research Fellow, Department of Pediatries, Agrigento; S. Grimaldi, Microcitemia Center, Crotone; B. Lanzone, Microcitemia Center, Legnago; L. Leardini, Department of Pediatrics, Biella; A. Mangiagli, Department of Pediatrics, Microcitemia Center, Siracusa; C. Melevendi, Department of Pediatrics, Galliera Hospital, Genoa; A. Meo, Department of Pediatrics, Microcitemia Service, University of Messina, Messina; W. Monguzzi, Department of Pediatrics, University of Milan, Monza; R. Naldini, Department of Pediatrics, Adria; A.M. Pasquino, Endocrinology Service, University of Rome, Rome; G. Ponzi, Department of Pediatrics, Casarano; G. Quarta, Microcitemia Center, Brindisi; A. Romondia, Department of Pediatrics, Foggia; L. Ruggiero, Department of Pediatrics, Lecce; A. Saviano, Department of Pediatrics, Cardarelli Hospital, Naples; M.F. Scarfia, Microcitemia Center, Caltanisetta; I. Stefano, Microcitemia Center, SS Annunziata Hospital, Taranto; G. Tamborino, Department of Pediatrics, Gallipoli; S. Terzoli, Department of Pediatrics, University of Milan, Milan

S. Andò et al. (Eds.)
Endocrine Disorders in Thalassemia
© Springer-Verlag Berlin Heidelberg 1995

whom were over the age of 15 years. By 1991, 36 centers were participating, treating a total of 3092 patients with thalassemia major and involving 38 physicians.

Results

Failure of puberty was the major clinical consequence of endocrine abnormalities present in 41% of boys and 39.5% of girls over the age of 15 years. Secondary amenorrhea was recorded in 26% of patients, primary hypothyroidism in 5.7% (mean age 15.7 years), insulin-dependent diabetes mellitus in 4.1% (mean age 17.6 years), and hypoparathyroidism in 3% (mean age 18.3 years). The incidences of hypothyroidism, insulin-dependent diabetes mellitus, and hypoparathyroidism differed in the different centers participating in the study, while the incidence of disorders of pubertal maturation was very similar.

Conclusion

Iron overload is always present in thalassemia major and it has been thought to be the cause of the endocrine abnormalities, [2]. This assumption is supported by histological studies of different endocrine glands [2, 5, 7]. The precise mechanism whereby iron overload causes tissue damage is not yet completely understood, although there is evidence for mechanisms such as free radical formation and lipid peroxidation resulting in mithochondrial, lysosomial, and sarcolemmal membrane damage.

It is difficult to compare our results with those reported in the literature, as studies involving as many patients as in our study have not been reported. In general, it seems that the prevalence of hypogonadism is similar [3], while the numbers of patients with primary hypothyroidism and diabetes mellitus are lower than those reported in the past [4, 5].

From our data it can be concluded that endocrine complications in thalassemic patients are fairly common. Therefore, periodic endocrine investigations should be carried out in patients with thalassemia major in order to detect those who require hormone replacement therapy.

References

1. Brezis M. Shalev O, Leibel B, Bernheim J, Ben-Ishay D (1980) Phosphorus retention and hypoparathyroidism associated with transfusional iron overload in thalassaemia. Miner Electrolyte Metab 4: 57–61
2. Costin G, Kogut M, Hyman CB, Ortega J (1979) Endocrine abnormalities in thalassaemia major. Am J Dis Child 133: 497–502
3. De Sanctis V, Vullo C, Katz M et al. (1989) Endocrine complications in thalassaemia major. In: Buckner CD, Gale RP, Lucarelli G (eds) Advances and controversies in thalassaemia therapy. Liss, New York; pp 77–83

4. Lassmann MN, Genel M, Wise JK, Hendler R, Felig P (1974) Carbohydrate homeostasis and pancreatic islet cell function in thalassaemia. Ann intem Med 80: 65–69
5. Rahier J, Loozen S, Goebbels RM, Abrrahem M (1987) The haematochromatic human pancreas: a quantitative immunohistochemical and ultrastructural study. Diabetologia 30: 5–12
6. Saudek CD, Hemm RM, Peterson CM (1977) Abnormal glucose tolerance in β-thalassemia major. Metabolism 26: 43–52
7. Suda K (1985) Hemosiderin deposition in the pancreas. Arch Pathol Lab Med 109: 996–999

Communications

Growth in Homozygous β-Thalassemic Patients

M. C. Galati, G. Raiola, P. Puzzonia, C. Consarino,
S. Grimaldi, S. Morgione, E. Santilli, R. Mancuso, A. Vero,
and S. Magro

Introduction

Advances in transfusion and chelation therapy have significantly increased the life expetancy of patients with homozygous β-thalassemia. However, a variety of endocrine abnormalities frequently occur in such patients. A number of studies have shown that as thalassemic patients approach the age of puberty, a percentage develop growth retardation [1]. The growth failure of these patients has been attributed to hypothyroidism, delayed sexual maturation, hypogonadism, zinc deficit, and desferrioxamine toxicity. The aim of the present investigation was to evaluate a possible role of the GHRH-GH-IGF-I axis dysfunction in growth failure in homozygouys β-thalassemia.

Patients and Methods

We studied 42 transfusion-dependent homozygous β-thalassemic patients, 28 male and 14 female, aged 10–18 years. They were submitted to a regular transfusion program in order to keep pretransfusional hemoglobin values between 10.5 and 11 g/dl; in all iron overload was prevented by daily subcutaneous desferrioxamine treatment of a dosage of 40 mg/kg body wt, 8–12 h overnight.

All the patients were euthyroid (mean serum TSH 3.50 ± 1.20 µU/ml; mean serum FT 41.68 ± 0.35 pmol/l; mean serum TBG 19.41 ± 3.8 µg/ml; intestinal malabsorption was excluded by measuring serum antibodies to gliadine and blood xilose concentration after oral load. Serum ferritin (n.r. 30–233 ng/ml), AST (n.r. 0–18 U/l) and ALT (n.r. 0–22 U/l) were also measured. All the patients were still in prepubertal stages according to Tanner's puberty staging and with prepubertal response of luteinzing hormone (LH) and follicle-stimulating hormone (FSH) to LH-releasing hormone (LHRH) stimulation.

Heigths were determined using a Harpenden stadiometer, growth velocity was calculated over a period of 12 months. Bone age was evaluated according to the TW2 method. Height and growth velocity were expressed as height standard deviation score (HSDS) and height velocity standard deviation score (HVSDS) compared with bone age according to Tanner.

In all patients basal plasma IGF 1 was measured by immunoradiometric assay after acid extraction (IRMA-catalog number DSL 5600). Basal plasma IGF 1 was mea-

S. Andò et al. (Eds.)
Endocrine Disorders in Thalassemia
© Springer-Verlag Berlin Heidelberg 1995

sured in 20 bone age and sex-matched healthy controls. In all patients basal plasma
GH was measured by RIA (hGH I kit RADIM catalog number KP 9).

All patients underwent an arginine Test; 0.5 g/kg body wt. was intravenously
infused over a period of 30 min; samples for GH assay were collected at 30, 0, 30,
60, 90, and 120 min after the end of infusion. Subjects with a GH response to the
arginine test below 10 ng/ml were submitted to a second GH stimulation test. At
first we chose the insulin test (i. v. bolus of 0.1 U/kg body wt.; blood was sampled
at 0, 15, 30, 45, 60, 75, and 90 min after injection); however, since this test was
disturbing for some patients, we used the clonidine test (an oral dose of 150 µg/m²
body surface area; samples were taken at 0, 30, 60, 90 and 120 min after clonidine
administration. These provocative GH tests were performed after priming with sex
steroids (ethinilestradiol 0.01 µg/day orally, given on 4 consecutive days to female
subjects; a single dose of 125 mg testosterone i.m. given 3 days before GH stimulation test to male subjects).

In patients with a GH response to a second pharmacological stimulation test
below 10 ng/ml á GHRH test and an IGF 1 generation test were performed. In this
case we faced a classic GH deficit and we wanted to localize the damage hypo-
talamic if GHRH-induced GH peak was more than 20 ng/ml; hypophyseal if less
than 20 ng/ml and determine which children might benefit from GH therapy. The
first test was carried out by intravenous injection of GHRH (1 µg/kg body wt.) and
blood was sampled at 0, 15, 30, 60, 90 and 120 min; a single oral dose of piridostig-
min (2 mg/kg body wt.) was given 60 min before the GHRH injection. The second
one was performed measuring basal plasma (GF) levels and IGFI response after
single daily doses of GH (0.1 U/kg body wt.) given on 4 consecutive days.

The patients who showed a GH response to insulin or clonidine greater than or
equal to 10 ng/ml underwent an IGFI generation test. As it was not possible at our
institution to assess spontaneous GH secretion, we used the 9-generation test as
predictive of response to GH treatment [4].

Basal plasma GH evaluation and an arginie stimulation test were performed in
15 bone age- and sex-matched healthy controls to calculate the normal GH peak
range. Statistical analysis included the calculation of means and standard deviations
by Student's test and analysis of variance.

Results

Auxoligical data are reported in Table 1 and 2. Compared with 20 bone age- and
sex-matched healthy controls, homozygous β-thalassemic patients showed significantly lower mean IgF1 levels (127 ± 90 versus 346 ± 105 ng/ml in male subjects
and 93 ± 37 versus 424 ± 105 in female subjects; significances: $p = 0$).

Basal serum GH levels did not differ significantly between patients and in controls
(4.46 ± 45 versus 1.9 ± 3.5 ng/ml). A repeated blunted GH response to conventional stimuli was found in three patients (one male, two female); the GHRH-induced
GH secretion was normal in all three cases.

A 13-year-old boy, M.M., had a height around the third percentile and a height
velocity below the third percentile; the IGFI response to GH stimulation was great-

Table 1. Auxological data of 28 male patients

Case no.	CA	Height (cm)	HSDS	HV (cm/y) 1990	HV (cm/y) 1992	HVSDS/BA 1990	HVSDS/BA 1992	BA (TW2) 1990	BA (TW2) 1992	DBA (months)
1	9.84	122.5	−2.3	6.1	5.2	−0.1	−1.7	6	7.78	−25
2	9.95	132.7	−0.7	5.1	4.4	−0.5	−1.1	8.25	10.13	2
3	11.40	139.7	−0.7	4	2.5	−1.9	−3.7	8.5	10.06	−16
4	11.76	142	−0.7	4.8	4.6	−0.3	−0.9	10.8	12.87	13
5	11.84	143.1	−0.6	3.9	1.5	−1.9	−5.2	9.5	10.96	−11
6	11.98	136.5	−1.5	5.3	5.3	0.4	0	10.8	12.61	4
7	12.75	149	−0.6	5.8	7.5	1.2	−0.1	11.25	13.37	7
8	12.91	147.1	−0.8	4.2	5.8	0.9	−2.5	11.8	13.6	8
9	13	141	−1.6	3.9	1.9	−2	−4.7	8.8	10.46	−30
10	13.20	148.5	−0.6	4.9	4.6	−0.4	−0.5	9.9	11.49	−21
11	13.22	142.2	−1.4	5.2	4.6	0	−0.5	9.7	11.46	−21
12	13.54	145	−1.4	5	8.5	−0.2	−0.6	12.35	14.14	7
13	13.54	142	−1.8	2.5	3.9	−3.6	−3.2	11.5	13.37	− 2
14	14.08	137	−2.8	3.5	2	−2.1	−4.9	11.5	13.23	−10
15	14.20	145.6	−1.8	5.8	5.7	0.8	0.1	9.9	11.13	−37
16	14.22	139.2	−2.6	4.4	4	−1.1	−1.5	9.15	10.93	−39
17	14.4	148.2	−1.9	3.8	3.5	−1.3	−4.5	11.7	13.52	−11
18	14.63	151.4	−1.5	4.8	7.2	−0.3	−1.8	12.1	13.64	−12
19	14.64	147.2	−2	3.8	3.2	−1.9	−3.3	12.7	14.64	0
20	14.76	141	−3.3	3	0.8	−2.4	−7.2	12.3	13.88	−11
21	14.76	142	−3.2	3.9	1.8	−1.3	−6.2	12.3	14.18	− 7
22	14.81	145	−2.8	4.4	3.1	−1.3	−4.3	12.7	14.56	− 3
23	15.56	137.3	−4.3	4.7	5.9	−0.4	−0.5	11.1	12.99	−31
24	15.75	143.2	−3.8	3.7	0.5	−1.9	5.4	10.75	12.56	−38
25	16.01	142	−4.5	3.6	3	−1.8	−5.3	12	13.83	−26
26	16.81	155.5	−2.8	4.2	4.2	−1.5	−2.4	12.9	14.74	−25
27	16.92	150.5	−3.6	4.4	2.3	−1.3	−4.1	13	14.86	−25
28	18.75	159	−2.4	3.4	1.8	−2.3	−5.4	12.8	14.43	−52

Table 2. Auxological data of 14 female patients

Case. no.	CA	Height (cm)	HSDS	HV (cm/y) 1990	HV (cm/y) 1992	HVSDS/BA 1990	HVSDS/BA 1992	BA (TW2) 1990	BA (TW2) 1992	DBA (months)
1	9.89	128	−1.33	5.4	4.2	−0.1	−1.5	8.7	10.37	6
2	9.92	137	0.1	5.6	5.9	−0.9	−2.2	11.1	11.96	24
3	10.90	130.2	−1.8	5.6	3	0.2	−3	8.4	10.69	− 2
4	10.99	135.2	−1.1	5	4.2	−0.6	−1.5	8.8	10.35	− 8
5	11.04	123.7	−2.7	5.4	4.2	−0.4	−1.6	7.2	9.14	−23
6	12.24	131.7	−2.3	4.7	3.2	−1	−2.8	8.2	9.64	−31
7	13.30	135	−3.5	4.9	2.1	−0.7	−4.9	9.5	11.29	−24
8	13.39	155	0.4	5.2	0	−2.2	−3.1	12.6	13.9	6
9	13.67	152.1	−0.9	3.6	1.7	−2.3	−5.8	9.7	11.44	−27
10	13.76	142.2	−2.7	6.6	5.8	0.7	−0.7	10.9	12.85	−11
11	13.78	139.9	−3.1	4.7	3.2	−0.9	−4.3	10.1	11.88	−23
12	13.91	134.8	−3.4	5.2	3.5	−0.4	−2.6	8.4	10.45	−41
13	15.38	155	−1.3	6.2	2.3	−1.6	−2.2	11.5	13.43	−23
14	15.79	138.5	−3.9	4.4	1.7	−2.1	−3.6	11.1	12.96	−34

Abbreviations: CA, age; DBA, delayed bone age:
HSDS, height standard deviation score; HV, growth velocity; HVSDS/BA, height velocity standard deviation score by bone age; TW 2, method for determining bone age

er than 100% compared with his basal IgF 1 level. Now he is the only one receiving GH treatment (0.1 U/kg/day, 6 days a week).

In the case of a 10-year-old girl, B. A., the height was around the 50th percentile, but up to a year ago the patient had grown to reach the 75th percentile; the IGFI generation test showed a poor response to GH stimulation.

Another girl, C. F., who was 13 years height had a around the 25th centile; she was the same as the year earlier, when she was in the 75th percentile; during the 12-month period her growth velocity was zero. This patient refused to undergo an IGFI generation test. In this case the GH response to arginine and clonidine was just below 10 ng/ml (7 and 9.1 ng/ml, respectively) and the girl had an increased body mass index (33.3 kg/m^2); since GH levels fall with increasing body mass [5], the GH response could appear to be subnormal.

In four male patients the GH peak was below 10 ng/ml during the first GH stimulation test and greater than 10 ng/ml during the second one. Only one patient agreed to undergo IGFI stimulation test, but he was a nonresponder.

In 35 patients the GH response to the arginine test was greater than 10 ng/ml, but in some of these it seemed to us excessive. For this reason an arginine GH stimulation test was performed in 15 bone age- and sex-matched healthy controls to calculate the normal GH peak range (mean = 23.9 ± 8.8 ng/ml; range = $6.3 - 41.5$ ng/ml). Thus, we were able to say that in 16 patients (nine male, seven female) the GH peak was abnormal (above the upper range of the value in the controls). All seven girls and five boys agreed to undergo an IGFI generation test and in all we found a poor response to GH administration.

No correlation was found between GH response to conventional stimuli and serum ferritin levels. All the patients studied had clinical and/or biochemical evidence of liver damage (mean serum AST = 95 31 U/l; mean serum ALT = 89 27 U/l).

Discussion

Historically, patients with homozygous β-thalassaemia show growth failure, mainly evident at the age of puberty; its dependence on defective GH secretion is not fully established [1-3]. Some authors have found a normal GH response to arginine, insulin, L-dopa, and GHRH, where as others have reported inadequate hormone release following different pharmacological challenges [6]. We found a repeated blunted GH response to conventional stimuli in three of 42 our patients. (7.1%). In these three cases we did not find delayed bone age, but a GH deficit in these patients could be acquired and, if recent, could be compatible with a normal bone age. Priming with sex steroids, performed before all the GH stimulation tests in all patients studied, enhances the GH responses in delayed puberty and thus makes the diagnosis of GH deficit more accurate. In 16 patients we found an excessive GH peak during the GH stimulation test. Previous studies in these patients had shown low plasma IGFI levels and poor increase in this peptide after 4 days of GH treatment [7]. We used the IGFI generation test as a selection criterion to predict which short children might benefit from GH therapy [4], although this predictive value is controversial and a GH-induced synthesis of IGFI by growth plate chondrocytes has been demostrated, suggesting a direct growth-promoting effect of GH on cartilage [8, 9]. In all the patients we found low basal plasma IGFI levels, and in all patients but one a poor or absent response to short-term GH administration. Liver failure might account for IGFI deficency or an IGFI-poor response to GH administration, and this would result in high GH levels [2]. However, the low IGFI levels and the impairment of GH secretion related to iron toxicity may play a role in the etiology of growth retardation in homozygous β-thalassemia.

References

1. Kattamis C, Touliatos M, Holdas S, Matsaniotis N (1979) Growth of children with thalassemia: effect of different transfusion regimens. Arch Dis Child 45: 502–505
2. Long RG (1980) Endocrine aspects of liver disease. Br Med 1: 225–228
3. Colombo A, Larizza D, Garibaldi E, Bozzola M, Gasparoni MC, Peretti L (1977) Crescita ed alcuni parametri endocrinologici con particolare riferimento al GH nella thalassemia major. Minerva Pediatr 29: 1235–1239
4. Rudman D, Moffitt SD, Blackston RD, Cushman RA, Bain RP, Patterson JH (1981) Children with normal variant short stature: treatment with human growth hormone for six months. N Engl J Med 305: 123–131
5. Bengtsson Ba, Brummer RJ, Basaeus N (1990) Growth hormone and body composition. Horm Res 33 {Suppl 4]: 19–24
6. Pintor C, Cella SG, Manso P, Corda R, Dessl C, Locatelli V, Muller EE (1986) Impaired growth hormone in thalassemia major. J Clin Endocrinol Metab 62: 263–267
7. Werther JA, Metthews RN, Burger HG, Herington AC (1981) Lack of response of nonsuppressible insulin-like activity to short-term administration of human growth hormone in thalassemia major. J Clin Endocrinol Metab 53: 806–809
8. Underwood LR, D'Ercole JA, Clemmons DR, Van Wyk JJ (1986) Paracrine functions of somato-medins. Clin Endocrinol Metab 15: 59–77
9. Werther GA, Haynes KM, Barnard R, Waters MJ (1990) Visual demonstration of growth hormone receptors on human growth plate chondrocytes. J Clin Endocrinol Metab 70: 1725–1731

Relationship Between GH Response to Stimuli, Levels of IGF-1, and Final Height

R. V. G. García-Mayor, L. F. Pérez Mendez, C. Páramo, R. Luna, and A. Andrade

Introduction

Intensive transfusion regimens have significantly improved the prognosis for patients with thalassemia major. However, growth failure and hypogonadism are still major problems. Growth failure is generally accepted as beginning at the age of 10, with a marked decline in the growth rate after the age of 12–14 years [1, 2]. A recent report shows that height impairment occurs before the age of 10 [3]. While it is possible that delayed puberty may be responsible for the failure to grow during the physiological period of puberty, factors determining precocious growth impairment are less clear.

Endocrine studies in young children have frequently, but not always, revealed the presence of a normal GH response to provocative stimuli. However, low plasma insulin-like growth factor-1 (IGF-1) activity was found in several studies [4, 5]. The aim of the present study was to investigate the relationship between GH response to pharmacological stimuli, the levels of IgF-1, and final height in thalassemic patients.

Subjects and Methods

Ten patients (six girls and four boys) with β-thalassemia major participated in a longitudinal study on endocrine abnormalities in thalassemia. The patients received blood transfusions to maintain hemoglobin levels above 10.5 g/dl and received chelation therapy with desferrioxamine, 40 mg/kg/day, over 8 h at night by subcutaneous pump, 5 days a week.

GH-provocative stimuli (clonidine 0.10 mg/m) were administered at prepubertal and pubertal stages of development. Serum IGF-1 (mean of three samples) was also determined at the same stages of development. Ten non obese subjects of normal height matched for sex and age with the patients served as a control group.

Height was measured with a Harpenden stadiometer. The height was evaluated according to Tanner's charts. GH was measured by IRMA using a commercial kit (Allegro-Nichols) and unextracted IGF-1 by RIA-DAB (Allegro-Nichols). The results of hormone tests were evaluated retrospectively in relation to the final height of the patients.

S. Andò et al. (Eds.)
Endocrine Disorders in Thalassemia
© Springer-Verlag Berlin Heidelberg 1995

Results

One of four children with short final height (SFH) and two of six with normal final height (NFH) had a GH peak clonidine stimulation under 10 ng/ml at the prepubertal stage. All children had a GH response to pharmacological stimulation above 10 ng/ml at the pubertal stage of development (Table 1). The mean values of GH peak in either prepubertal or pubertal stages were not significantly different between SFH and NFH groups of patients (Table 1).

No significant difference with respect to mean IGF-1 levels at prepubertal and pubertal stages was observed between the NFH group of patients and the control group (0.93 ± 0.25 and 2.5 ± 1.24 U/ml for prepubertal and pubertal stages, respectively). The mean values of IGF-1 in both prepubertal and pubertal stages of development were significantly lower in the SFH group than in the NFH group (Table 1).

In the SFH group, three of four pubertal children and all prepubertal children show IGF-1 levels under the reference values.

Discussion

The present data indicate that GH deficiency is not a principal cause of growth failure in thalassemic children, in agreement with earlier reports [4, 5]. Moreover, the lack of concordance between the results of the GH-provocative test and the serum IGF-1 levels suggests that abnormalities in IGF-1 generation by the liver [6]

Table 1. GH after stimulation peak and IGF-1 levels at prepubertal and pubertal stages of development

Patient	Sex	Prepubertal GH peak (ng/ml)	IGF-1 (U/ml)	Pubertal GH peak (ng/ml)	IGF-1 (U/ml)
			SHF Group		
VPV	M	21.5	0.31	36.0	0.75
JCF	M	6.1	0.28	125.0	0.07
MCT	M	20.5	0.30	22.0	0.31
PCL	F	10.2	0.40	30.6	0.38
		14.5	0.32	25.2	0.37
		$\pm$ 7.5	± 0.05	± 10.2	± 0.28
			NFH Group		
CZG	M	4.1	0.80	12.0	1.60
MPV	F	12.0	0.80	20.0	1.22
FUD	F	11.1	0.65	14.0	1.77
SFC	F	8.4	0.60	16.0	1.90
RZG	F	22.5	0.80	29.0	2.20
MFC	F	10.2	0.95	22.0	3.30
		11.4	0.76*	18.8	1.99**
		$\pm$ 6.1	± 0.12	$\pm$ 6.2	± 0.75

*$p < 0.05$, **$p < 0.01$

or the so-called GH neurosecretory dysfunction [7] could explain the prepubertal growth failure in some children with β-thalassemia major.

Also, our results suggest that the determination of serum IGF-1 levels could have prognostic value for final height in thalassemic children.

References

1. Bogna-Pignatti C, De Stefano P, Zonta L, Villo C, De Sanctis V, Melevendi C, Naselle A, Masera G, Terzoli S, Gabitti V, Piga A (1985) Growth and sexual maturation in thalassemia major. J Pediatr 106: 150–155
2. Kattamis C, Liakopoulus T, Kattamis A (1990) Growth and development in children with thalassemia major. Acta Paediatr Scand [Suppl] 366: 111–117
3. Cavallo L, De Mattia D, Giobbe T, Liuzzi S, Aquafreda A, Sabato V, Schettini F (1991) Growth in homozigous beta-thalassemic patients. In: Cavallo L, Job J, New MI, (Eds) Serono symposia. Raven New York, pp 47–54
4. Masala A, Meioni T, .Gallisani D, Alagna S, Rovassio PP, Rassau S, Milia F (1984) Endocrine functioning in multitransfused prepubertal patients with homozygous beta thalassemia. J Clin Endocrinol Metab 58: 667–670
5. Leger J, Girot R, Crosnier H, Postel-Vinay MC, Rappaport R (1989) Normal growth hormone response to growth hormone releasing hormone in children with thalassemia major before puberty: a possible age-related effect. J Clin Endocrinol Metab 69: 453–456
6. Herington AC, Werther GA, Mattews RN, Burger HGH (1981) Studies on the possible mechanism for deficiency of nonsuppressible insulin-like activity in thalassemia major. J Clin Endocrinol Metab 52: 393–398
7. Caruso-Nicoletti M, Mancuso M, Spadaro G, Lo Presti D, Di Gregorio F, Reitano G (1991) Twelve-hour growth hormone secretion in thalassemic patients. In: Cavallo L, Job J, New MI, (eds) Serono symposia. Raven New York pp 249–252

Growth Hormone Secretion in Thalassemic Patients

M. Caruso-Nicoletti, G. Tinnirello, V. Panebianco, M. Mancuso,
G. Spadaro, D. Lo Presti, and F. Di Gregorio

Introduction

During the past 10 years significant achievements have been made in the treatment
of β-thalassemia major. Nevertheless, the improved survival of these patients has
led to the appearance of several complications, which now represent the major clinical problems in the disease. Endocrine disorders are very common, and growth failure is one of the most frequent. Short stature is present in approximately 30% of
our thalassemic patients ($n = 200$). However, the pathogenesis of the growth disturbances of thalassemic patients has not yet been elucidated. The role of growth hormone (GH) deficiency in the growth impairment of these patients is controversial.
Hence, we have studied GH secretion in a group of thalassemic patients with short
stature.

Patients and Methods

We have studied 31 patients with homozygous β-thalassemia. All patients had been
on a transfusion regimen with packed red cells since approximately 1 year of age.
Pretransfusion hemoglobin concentration was always mantained at > 10.5 g%. In
addition, they had received deferoxamine (50 mg/kg/day) 6 days a week since
1979. Compliance to chelation therapy was acceptable in all of them. The patients
age range was 10.7–19.5 years; all of them exhibited short stature ($<$ 3rd percentile), reduced growth velocity ($<$ 10th percentile), and delayed bone age. Clinical
and auxological characteristics of the patients are shown in Table 1. Bone age was
evaluated according to the TW2 method [1]. Height was measured with a Harpen-

Table 1. Clinical and auxological characteristics of the patients

Patients	M/F	Mean ± SD
Prepubertal	8/8	
Pubertal	1/2	
On sex steroid therapy	10/2	
Age (years)		13.8 ± 2.3
Bone age (SDS)		-1.8 ± 1.2
Height (SDS)		-2.7 ± 0.8
Growth velocity (cm/year)	3.1 ± 1.0	

S. Andò et al. (Eds.)
Endocrine Disorders in Thalassemia
© Springer-Verlag Berlin Heidelberg 1995

den stadiometer. Both bone age and height were expressed as standard deviation scores (SDS) according to Tanner and Whitehouse [2]. GH secretion was evaluated by an arginine-insulin test ($n = 12$), seven patients were submitted to priming with sex steroids before GH testing, three did not undergo the priming, and two were tested both before and after priming. In addition, spontaneous GH secretion was assessed using a continuous withdrawal pump [3] in seven patients. Blood was collected from 8 p.m. to 8 a.m. During this time the children slept spontaneously for 8 h. The mean 12-h concentration of GH (MGHC) was measured in the sample obtained. Thyroid hormone levels were measured in all patients.

Results

All patients were euthyroid; four of them were receiving thyroid hormone replacement therapy. We considered those patients who exhibited a peak GH level > 10 ng/ml to at least one stimulus as responders to AITT. All except five patients exhibited normal response to the AITT. However, three of them were those who had not undergone to sex steroid priming. The two patients who were tested both before and after priming did not show a positive response the first time but they did the second time. MGHC was normal (> 4 ng/ml) in three patients and low in four of them; two of these patients were also non-responders to the AITT.

Discussion

The growth impairment observed in thalassemic patients is probably a complication of an intensive transfusion regimen (hemocromatosis) and/or chelation thereapy. Several factors have been considered to play a role in the growth disturbances of thalassemic patients: zinc deficiency [4], the toxic effect of deferoxamine [5], and hemocromatosis-induced GH deficiency [6], as well as a reduction of IGF-1 production from the liver [7]. In addition, recent studies have suggested the possibility of a hypothalamic-pituitary dysfunction [8, 9]. We have studied stimulated GH secretion in 31 short thalassemic patients and spontaneous GH secretion in seven of them in order to evaluate the role of GH deficiency and/or neurosecretory dysfunction in their growth failure. We found a normal GH response to provocative tests in the great majority of these patients. In addition, among the five patients with abnormal GH response, three would probably have responded if they had been submitted to sex steroid priming, as suggested by the results in the two patients who were tested both before and after priming. Therefore, we think that GH deficiency is not frequent among short thalassemic patients, and when present, in most cases it is secondary to delayed puberty. Indeed, impairment of sexual development is even more frequent than short stature in thalassemic patients [10]. Spontaneous GH secretion was low in four of seven patients, and in two of them this finding was associated with normal response to the stimulation test, suggesting a neurosecretory dysfunction, as reported previously [9]. The mechanism underlying the hypothalamic-pituitary dysfunction in thalassemic patients has to be elucidated.

In conclusion, the results of this study support the hypothesis that classic GH deficiency is not the cause of short stature in thalassemic patients. Further studies are needed to establish whether spontaneous GH secretion is impaired in a large percentage of these patients and whether they could benefit from GH therapy.

References

1. Tanner JM, Whitehouse RH, Marshall WA, Healy MJR, Goldstein H (1975) Assessment of skeletal maturity and prediction of adult height (TW2 method). Academic, London
2. Tanner JM, Whitehouse RH (1976) Clinical and longitudinal standards for height, weight, height velocity, weight velocity and stages of puberty. Arch Dis Child 51: 170–179
3. Kowarski A, Thompson RG, Migeon CJ, Blizzard RM (1971) Determination of integrated plasma concentration and true secretion rate of human growth hormone. J Clin Endocrinol Metab 32: 356–360
4. Arcasoy A, Cavdar AC (1975) Changes in trace minerals (serum iron, zinc, copper and magnesium) in thalassemia. Acta Haematol (Basel) 53: 341–346
5. De Virgilis S, Congia M, Frau F, Argiolu F, Diana G, Cucca F, Varsi A, Sanna G, Podda G, Fodde M, Pirastu FGF, Cao A (1988) Deferoxamine-induced growth retardation in patients with thalassemia major. J Pediatr 113: 661–669
6. Rivolta MR, De Micheli A, Capra M, Gelosa M, Lange E, Monguzzi W (1987) Growth hormone response to hypoglycemic stress in thalassemia major (Abstr). J Endocrinol Invest 10 [Suppl] 4: 84
7. Saenger P, Schwartz E, Markenson AL, Graziano JH, Levine LS, New MI, Hilgartner MW (1980) Depressed serum somatomedin activity in beta-thalassemia. J Pediatr 96: 214–218
8. Pintor C, Cella S, Manso P, Corda R, Dessi C, Locatelli V, Muller EE (1986) Impaired growth hormone (GH) response to GH-releasing hormone in thalassemia major. J Clin Endocrinol Metab 62: 263–267
9. Shehadeh N, Hazan A, Rudolf MCJ, Peleg I, Benderly A, Hochberg Z (1990) Neurosecretory dysfunction of growth hormone secretion in thalassemia major. Acta Paediatr Scand 79: 790–795
10. Borgna-Pignatti C, De Stefano P, Zonta L, Vullo C, De Sanctis V, Melevendi C, Naselli A, Masera G, Terzoli S, Gabutti V, Piga A (1985) Growth and sexual maturation in thalassemia major. J Pediatr 106: 150–155

Binding of Insulin-like Growth Factor-1
to Erythrocytes in Children with Thalassemia

M. Theochari, L. Stamogiannou, A. Kafourou, E. Spanos,
H. Nounopoulos, A. Bouloukos, and C. S. Bartsocas

Introduction

Short stature is a common feature of children with thalassemia [1–5]. Several studies have shown that when patients with thalassemia approach puberty they present a significant delay of growth [6, 7].

It has been observed that there is an inhibition in the growth rate after the first decade. These children do not achieve the acceleration of growth rate which occurs in prepubertal age in normal individuals.

The exact mechanism of the delayed physical growth of children with thalassemia has not yet been fully clarified. Various studies have shown normal response of growth hormone secretion in stimulation tests [2, 8–10] as well as a normal number of GH receptors [11]. Normal binding of GH by the hepatic receptors has also been shown [2, 11]. As a natural consequence, the interest of many investigators was directed towards the activity of somatomedins in thalassemia. It is known that somatomedins A and C are identical to the insulin-like growth factor (IGF-1) which is a polypeptide with promotion activity and which is quite similar to human insulin in respect to its aminoacid sequence, structure, and biological activity. IGF-1 factor, as a mediator of growth hormone action, depends on GH levels [12] and acts through its own receptors, which are present in many types of cells and tissues. The exact function of the IGF-1 receptors has not been fully clarified, but they have been proved to be responsible for the anabolic and replicating response of the cells to IGF-1.

We had observed previously that IGF-1 levels were reduced in thalassemic children [13]. Similar findings have been reported by other authors, too [3, 9]. The above results prompted us to study IGF-1 and its receptors in our patients.

Material and Methods

Fourteen children (six boys and eight girls) aged 4–15 years with homozygous β-thalassemia were studied and compared with ten healthy controls of the same age and sex. All were at Tanner pubertal stage 1. Blood was always collected in the morning, before transfusion, in heparinized tubes.

The specific binding of IGF-1 in the erythrocytes of thalassemic children was measured with the RIA method. For the calculation the ^{125}I-Thr^{59}-IGF-1 analogue

S. Andò et al. (Eds.)
Endocrine Disorders in Thalassemia
© Springer-Verlag Berlin Heidelberg 1995

was used. The isolation of erythrocytes was performed by the method of Boyum [14]. A total of 400 µl of erythrocytes were incubated at 40 °C for 18–24 h with 50 µl of ^{125}I-Thr^{59}-IGF-1 (20000–30000 cpm) alone or with the addition of unlabeled IGF-1 analogue at concentrations varying between 2.5 and 160 ng/ml. The final volume was 500 µl. After incubation, duplicate 200 µl aliquots of suspension were layered over 200 µl of cold 2% BSA Hepes buffer in plastic microtubes. After microcentrifugation in a Sorvall RC 2-B Microfuge, supernatants were discarded and the radioactivity of the pellets was measured. Nonspecific binding was defined as that radioactivity that remained in the presence of 1 µg/ml of IGF analogue and was subtracted from the total binding determination to yield specific binding. Nonspecific binding was $8.9 \pm 0.4\%$ (mean $\pm$ SEM) of the total radioactivity added. Results were normalized to 3×10^9 cell/ml. The receptors of IGF-1 per cell (Ro) were calculated by the formula [15]:

$$Ro = \frac{\text{IGF-1-specific binding} \times 6.02 \times 10^{23}}{\text{Cell concentration}/1}$$

The measurements were carried out in the Biochemistry Laboratory, University of Athens. The statistical analysis was performed using Student's t-test.

Results

The IGF-1-specific binding by erythrocytes was found to be decreased in thalassemic children (9.51 ± 2.94) as compared with the controls (16.4 ± 0.29; $p < 0.05$). It was also observed that the number of IGF-1 receptors per erythrocyte was decreased (65.37 ± 24.66) in relation to those of healthy children (104.96 ± 1.86) with a statistically significant difference ($p < 0.05$). The IGF-1 values were found to be   lower in thalassemic children (0.70 ± 0.34) in relation to the controls (1.51 ± 0.60; $p < 0.001$). Results are shown in Table 1. The correlation between IGF-1 levels and the ^{125}I-IGF-1-specific binding was not statistically significant. Obviously this is due to the small number of patients and controls.

Table 1. Comparison of the ^{125}I-IGF-1 specific binding, IGF-1 receptors, and IGF-1 in the serum between patients and controls

	n	^{125}I-IGF-1-specific binding (%)	No. binding sites/ erythrocyte	IGF-1 (U/ml)
Controls	10	16.4 ± 0.29	104.96 ± 1.86	1.51 ± 0.60
Thalassemic children	14	9.51 ± 2.94	65.37 ± 24.66	0.70 ± 0.34
p		≤ 0.05	≤ 0.05	≤ 0.001

Discussion

Short stature constitutes a frequent problem in children with thalassemia [1–5]. The exact cause remains obscure. It is likely a result of interaction of several factors. Kattamis et al. [5] refer to three probable factors affecting growth: (a) the genotype, (b) the individual response to treatment, and (c) the complications of the disease and/or treatment.

Recently, endocrinologic studies have been directed towards the growth hormone–Sm axis and the receptors of these hormones. Most studies have proved that stimulation tests of GH in children with thalassemia are normal and that the secreted molecules of GH are immunologically and biologically active [2, 8–10]. It is known that liver is the main organ producing IGF-1 [16, 17]. The secondary hemosiderosis which appears in many organs, including liver, of patients with thalassemia may decrease the IGF-1 activity [3]. We observed in a previous study that IGF-1 levels are related more to the ferritin values than to the liver damage-hence, there may be a special inhibiting influence of the iron upon IGF-1 production.

In the past, specific and nonspecific inhibitors of IGF-1 have been reported in patients with malnutrition [18] and with chronic renal failure [19]. No IGF-1 inhibitors were found in patients' blood which could have explained the IGF-1 reduced activity [3, 9].

It is well known that IGF-1 receptors exist in various tissues [20] such as: fibroblasts [21–23], mononuclear cells [24–26], ovaries, brain, liver, placenta, and the erythrocytes [27, 28]. The erythrocytes may not be the most appropriate tissue for the study of IGF-1 receptors, as regards thalassemic children, but they are the most convenient and accessible for well-known reasons: (a) biopsy is unnecessary, (b) there is no need to draw a large quantity of blood for isolation of the mononuclear cells, and (c) human erythrocytes are easily isolated and studied [29–32].

Recent investigations have shown that the specific binding activity of IGF-1 by the erythrocytes was increased in healthy children of prepubertal age, when compared with adults, despite the normal levels of IGF-1 in both groups [33]. This fact may help to explain the accelerated growth in young people.

It is worth adding that Morris and coworkers [33] studied the effect of erythrocyte age upon the IGF-1-specific binding and found that there was no correlation with the reticulocytes. The same is also reported by Hizuka et al. [34].

The reduced activity of IGF-1 in thalassemia has been described by several investigators [3, 9]. These findings agree with our findings as well as with those of our previous study, where the IGF-1 levels were low in the serum of patients.

The present study confirms the view that the dysfunction of IGF-1 in children with thalassemia may be one of the reasons for short stature. This is also supported by the observations of Van Obberghen-Schiling et al. [22], Bierich et al. [23], and Morris et al. [33], who suppose that the resistance of the IGF-1 with decreased IGF-1 binding is likely to be the underlying cause of short stature in several disorders and possibly in children with β-thalassemia. Our study confirms this possibility on account of the decreased specific binding.

Further studies of the factors affecting receptor activity, binding protein, and IGF-1 are necessary in order to elucidate the cause of decreased growth of thalassemic children.

References

1. Kuo B, Zains E, Roginsky M (1968) Endocrine function in thalassemia major. J Clin Endocrinol Metab 28: 805–808
2. Lassmann MN, O'Brien RT, Pearson HA, Wise JK, Donabedian RK, Felig P, Genel M (1974) Endocrine evaluation in thalassemia major. Ann NY Acad Sci 232: 226-237
3. Saenger P, Schwartz E, Markenson AL, Graziano JH, Levine LS, New MT, Hilgartner MW (1980) Depressed serum somatomedin activity in β-thalassemia. J Pediatr 96: 214
4. Gabutti V, Piga A, Davico S et al. (1985) Evaluation and prevention of iron overload in thalassemic children. In: Sirchia G, Zanella A (eds) Thalassemia today. Centro Transfusionale Ospedale Maggiore Policlinico di Milano, Milan pp 95–100
5. Kattamis C, Liakopoulou T, Kattamis A (1990) Growth and development in children with thalassemia major. Acta Paediatr Scand [Suppl] 366: 111–117
6. Modell B, Berdoukas V (1984) The clinical approach to thalassemia. Grune and Stratton, London
7. Borgna-Pignatti C, De Stefano P, Zonta L et al. (1985) Growth and puberty in thalassemia major. In: Sirchia G, Zanella A (eds) Thalassemia today. Centro Transfusionale Ospedale Maggiore Policlinico di Milano, Milan, 89–92
8. Werther GA, Matthews RN, Burger HG, Herington AC (1981) Deficiency of non-suppressible insulin-like activity in thalassemia major. Arch Dis Child 56: 855–859
9. Herington AC, Werther GA, Matthews RN, Burger HG (1981) Studies on the possible mechanism for deficiency of nonsuppressible insulin-like activity in thalassemia major. Endocrinol Metab 52: 393–398
10. Canale VC, Steinherz P, New MJ, Erlandson M (1974) Endocrine function in thalassemia major. Ann NY Acad Sci 232: 333–345
11. Postel-Vinay MC, Girot R, Leger J, Hocquette JF, McKelvine P, Amar-Costesec A, Rappaport R (1989) No evidence for a defect in growth hormone binding to liver membranes in thalassemia major. Endocrinol Metab 68: 94–98
12. Philips LS, Vassilopoulou-Sellin R (1980) Somatomedins. II N Engl J Med 302: 438–446
13. Stamogiannou L, Siondi E, Kafourou A, Siafas K, Bouloukos T, Bartsocas C (1991) Receptors of SM-C in erythrocytes in children with thalassemia. 29th Panhellenic Pediatric Congress, May, 25–26 Crete
14. Boyum (1980) Separation of leukocytes from blood and bone marrow. Isolation of mononuclear cells and granulocytes from human blood. Scand J Clin Invest 21 [Suppl] 97: 77–89
15. Wajchenberg BL, Lerario AC, El-Andere W, Ohunuma LY, Toledo E, Souza JT (1984) Human erythrocyte insulin receptors in normal male and female subjects. Clin Endocrinol (Oxf) 20: 23–30
16. Philips LS, Herington AC, Karl IE, Daughaday WH (1976) Comparison of somatomedin activity in perfusates of normal and hypophysectomized rat livers with and without added growth hormone. Endocrinology 98: 606–614
17. Schalch DS, Heinrich VE, Drazin B, Johnson CJ, Miller LL (1979) Role of the liver in regulating somatomedin activity: hormonal effects on the synthesis and release of insulin-like growth factor and its carrier protein by the isolated prefused rat liver. Endocrinology 104: 1143–1151
18. Hintz RL, Suskind R, Amatayakul K, Thanangkul O, Olson R (1978) Plasma somatomedin and growth hormone values in children with protein-calorie malnutrition. J Pediatr 92: 153–156
19. Takano K, Hall K, Kastru KW, Hizuka N, Shizume K, Kawai K, Akimoto M, Takumo T, Sugino N (1979) Serum somatomedin A in chronic renal failure. J Clin Endocrinol Metab 48: 371–376
20. Nissley SP, Rechler MM (1984) Somatomedin/insulin-like growth factors tissue receptors. Clin Endocrinol Metab 13: 43–47

21. Rechler MM, Nissley SP, Podskalny JM, Moses AC, Fryklund L (1977) Identification of receptor for somatomedin-like polypeptide in human fibroblasts. J Clin Endocrinol Metab 44: 820–831
22. Van Obberghen-Schiling EE, Rechler MM, Romanus JA, Knight AB, Nissley SP, Humbel RE (1981) Receptors for insulin-like growth factor-1 are defective in fibroblasts cultured from a patient with leprechaunism. J Clin Invest 68: 1356–1365
23. Bierich JR, Moeller H, Ranke MB, Rosenfeld RG (1984) Pseudopituitary dwarfism due to resistance to somatomedin: a new syndrome. Eur J Pediatr 142-186
24. Thorsson AV, Hintz RL (1977) Specific ^{125}somatomedin receptor on circulating human mononuclear cells. Biochem Biophys Res Commun 74: 1566–1573
25. Rosenfeld R, Thorsson AV, Hintz RL (1979) Increased somatomedin sites in newborn circulating mononuclear cells. J Clin Endocrinol Metab 48: 456–461
26. Rosenfeld RG, Kemp SF, Gaspich S, Hintz RL (1981) In vivo modulation of somatomedin receptor sites: effects of growth hormone treatment of hypopituitary children. J Clin Endocrinol Metab 52: 759–764
27. Gambhir KK, Archer JA, Bradley CJ (1978) Characteristics of human erythrocyte insulin receptors. Diabetes 27: 701–708
28. Polychronakos C, Guyda HS, Posner BJ (1983) Receptors for the insulin-like growth factors on human erythrocytes. J Clin Endocrinol Metab 57: 436–438
29. Rinderknecht E, Humbel RE (1978) The amino acid sequence of human-like growth factor-1 (SM-C/IGF-1) receptor on cultured human fibroblast monolayers: regulation of receptor concentrations by SM-C/IGF-1 and insulin. J Clin Endocrinol Metab 55: 434
30. Wachslicht-Rodbard H, Muggeo M, Kahn CR, Saviolakis GA, Harrison LC, Flier JS (1981) Heterogeneity of the insulin receptor interaction in lipoatrophic diabetes. J Clin Endocrinol Metab 52: 416–425
31. Dons RF, Ryan J, Gorden P, Wachslicht-Rodbard H (1981) Erythrocyte and monocyte insulin binding in man: a comparative analysis in normal and disease states. Diabetes 30: 896–902
32. Massague J, Czech MP (1982) The subunit structures of two distinct receptors for the insulin-like growth factors I and II and their relationship to the insulin receptor. J Biol Chem 257: 5038–5045
33. Morris AM, Joyce JD, Reiter EO (1989) Increased insulin-like growth factor I binding to red blood cells of normal prepubertal children. Paediatr Res 25 4: 409–413
34. Hizuka N, Takano K, Tanaka J, Honda N (1985) Characterization of insulin-like growth factor I receptor on human erythrocytes. J Clin Endocrinol Metab 61: 1066–1070

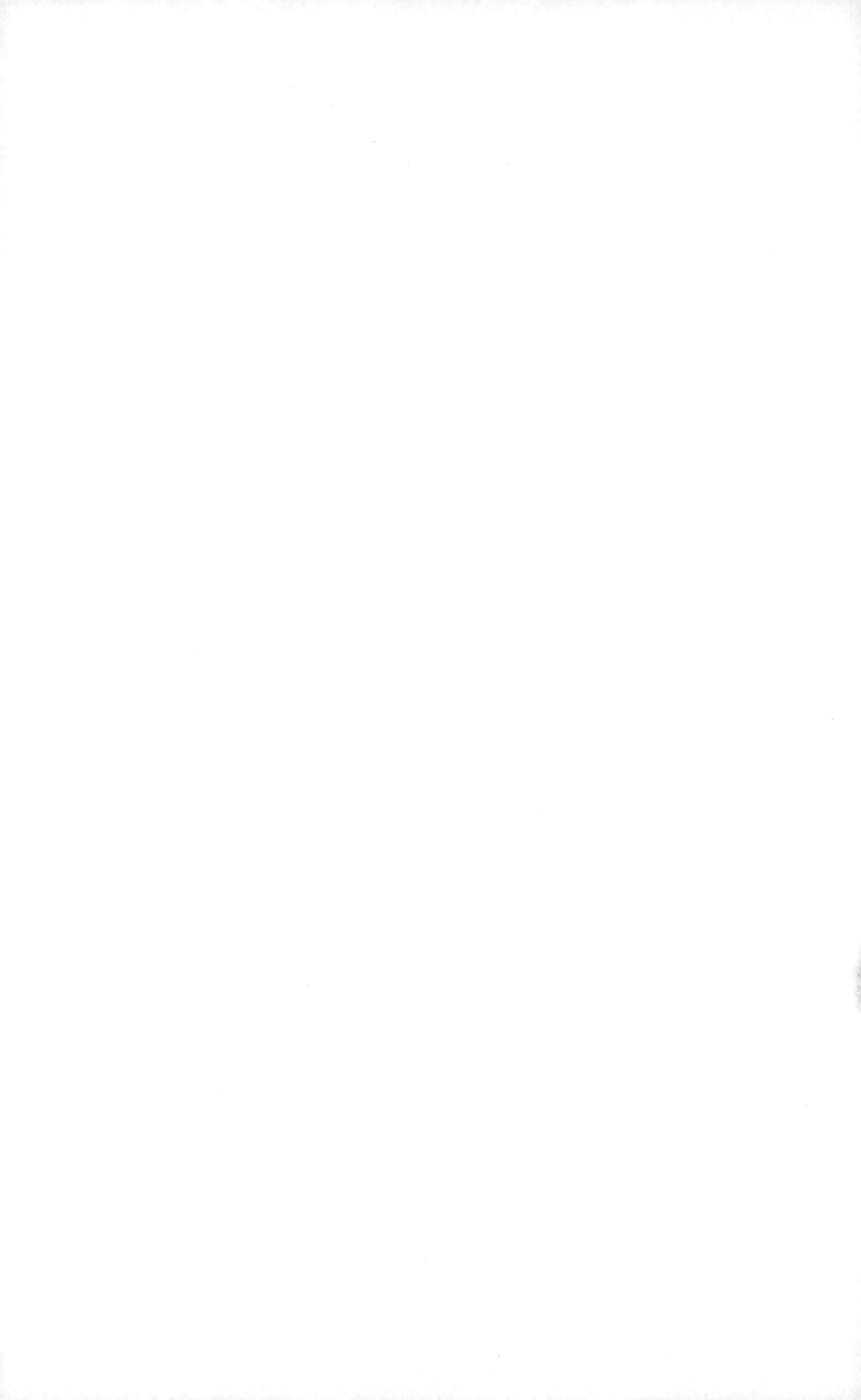

Evaluation of Thyroid Function in Thalassemic Patients Undergoing Long-term Blood Transfusion and Iron-Chelation Therapy

L. Pitrolo, C. Lo Pinto, P. D'Angelo, R. Malizia, and F. Lo Iacono

Introduction

Remarkable advances in blood transfusion and iron-chelation therapy have improved and prolonged the survival of patients with thalassemic syndromes. Because of this increase in mean survival, new therapeutic strategies have been designed in order to limit the most important complications involving heart, liver and endocrine tissues. Endocrine disorders are rarely reported as cause of death in thalassemics but they can worsen the quality of life of these patients. Most authors have reported high incidence of endocrine abnormalities in thalassemics and the iron overload is frequently indicated as the most important pathogenetic factor [1]. De Sanctis et al. [2], in a multicenter study, reported that endocrine abnormalities involve more than 50% of thalassemic patients. Particularly the incidence of thyroid disorders has shown a large variability, according to the findings reported in the various studies [3–5]. The aim of this study was to evaluate the thyroid function in 58 thalassemic patients in order to evaluate possible correlations with age, serum ferritin values, and liver impairment.

Patients and Methods

Fifty-eight transfusion-dependent thalassemic patients 31 female, 27 male with a median age of 19 years (range 5–44 years) were studied; 34 of them had been splenectomized. All patients received blood transfusions to maintain hemoglobing values $> 9.5–10$ g/dl, and desferrioxamine by subcutaneous infusion at a dose of 40–50 mg/kg/day, 5–6 times a week. The compliance to iron-chelation therapy was good (performed 5–7 times a week) in 63.7%. Serum thyroxine (T4), free-T4 (fT4), triiodothyroxine (T3), free-T3 (fT3), thyroid-stimulating hormone (TSH), and serum ferritin were measured by radioimmunologic assay (RIA). In all patients a TRH test was performed measuring TSH release before and 20, 60, 90, and 120 min after a standard administration of TRH (200 µg i.v.). Liver impairment was determined by serum level measurement of transaminases (ALT and AST). Statistical analysis was performed using the chi-square test, the linear correlation of Pearson, and the rank correlation test of Spearman and Kendall.

S. Andò et al. (Eds.)
Endocrine Disorders in Thalassemia
© Springer-Verlag Berlin Heidelberg 1995

Results

On physical examination none of our patients presented with clear clinical signs or symptoms of hypothyroidism. Of the 58 patients, seven had thyroid dysfunction (12%): two of them (3.4%) showed an uncompensated hypothyroidism and five (8.6%) a compensated hypothyroidism confirmed by an abnormal TRH test.

One of the two patients with uncompensated hypothyroidism, both aged 19 years, died some months later of severe cardiac failure due to a pre-existent dilatative miocardiopathy; the death was preceded by two other endocrine complications: diabetes and hypoparathyroidism. The other patients showed a symptomatic cardio-megal – probably due to hypothyroidism and iron overload without clear signs of heart failure, which strongly improved after the start of substitutive therapy with L-thyroxine (Eutirox Bracco). None of the five patient with compensated hypo-thyroidism had clinical signs of thyroid disorder (Table 1); they were between 14 and 42 years of age (median 22.2) and presented no other endocrine disorders. Clinical characteristics ot the patients with hypothyroidism are listed in Table 2.

None of the remaining 51 patients had an abnormal TRH test. Twenty of our patients presented with liver impairment, with serum transaminases AST and ALT twice the normal values. Serum ferritin levels were > 1000 ng/ml in 53 patients and > 4000 ng/ml in 15 of them (Table 3). On statistical analysis, we found a negative correlation between age and serum levels of T3 and fT3 ($p = 0.039$). Strangely, T3 and fT3 values were positively correlated with serum ferritin levels

Table 1. Serum levels of thyroid hormone and TSH in the five patients with compensated hypothyroidism

Patient	Age (years)	T3a	T4a	fT3a	fT4a	TSHa
1	19	2.0	80	4.5	11	6.0
2	20	2.0	46	3.0	7.8	54
3	42	0.5	52	3.3	8.7	12.6
4	14	1.2	73	4.8	7.8	10
5	16	1.1	82	3.7	9.7	10.5

Normal values: T3 = 0.6–2.1 nmol/l; T4 = 45–120 nmol/l; fT3 = 2.2–5.5 pmol/l; fT4 = 7.8–19.4 pmol/l; TSH = 0.2–4.0 µU/l.

Table 2. Clinical characteristics of patients with uncompensated (1–2) and compensated (3–7) hypothyroidism

Patient	Age (years)	Sex	Pubertal status	Diabetes	Hepatopathy	Cardiopathy	Splenectomy
1	19	F	3	yes	no	yes	no
2	19	M	2	yes	yes	yes	yes
3	20	F	4	no	yes	no	yes
4	42	M	3	no	no	yes	no
5	14	F	4	no	no	no	no
6	16	M	3	no	no	no	no
7	19	F	4	no˙	yes	no	yes

Table 3. Serum levels of thyroid hormone, TSH, ALT, and ferritin in our patients (values are expressed as mean +/– SD)

	Age (mean)	T3 (nmol/l)	T4 (nmol/l)	TSH (µU/l)	fT3 (pmol/l)	fT4 (pmol/l)	ALT (U/l)	Ferritin (ng/ml)
Normal patients (n = 51)	20.5	1.8 ± 0.5	83.6 ± 21.6	1.7 ± 0.8	4.1 ± 0.8	12.4 ± 2.7	79.6 ± 65.7	31.50 ± 19.39
Hypothyroid patients (n = 7)	21.2	1.2 ± 0.6	49.6 ± 30.6	48.3 ± 56	3.2 ± 1.4	6.1 ± 3.8	85.4 ± 38.8	22.95 ± 830.9

($p = 0.047$), and a strong correlation was found between serum ferritin levels and AST/ALT values. No correlation was seen between serum ferritin levels and hypothyroidism.

Discussion

Hypothyroidism is a frequent endocrine disorder of thalassemic patients. A review of the literature showed a prevalence of between 3 and 34.7%, according to various studies reported [2, 3, 5, 6]. We found a low incidence of uncompensated (3.4%) and compensated hypothyroidism (8.6%) in our patients. All showed characteristics of primary hypothyroidism and the median age was 21.2 years. According to the data in the literature, there is no correlation between high levels of serum ferritin and thyroid dysfunction; the role of iron overload as a cause of hypothyroidism remains controversial. The results reported by De Sanctis et al. [2] support iron-chelation therapy for the improvement of thyroid function in thalassemic patients, especially in subclinical hypothyroidism, underlining the pathogenetic role of iron overload in thyroid dysfunction.

No correlation has been found between serum levels of T3 and T4 and liver damage. From the data in the literature, it is known that hepatic dysfunction can be responsible for hypothyroidism because of decreased extrathyroid transformation of T4 in to T3 by T4-5-hepatic dejodasis. Although 34.4% of patients presented with conspicuous liver damage, we did not detect any significant correlation between levels of transaminases and thyroid dysfunction. Other factors may play a role in reducing thyroid function in thalassemic patients. Chronic hypoxia, both before diagnosis and in the first years of treatment (especially for older patients) can be an important factor in determining thyroid damage [5]. This was indirectly confirmed by our patients who showed a strong correlation between older age and reduction of serum levels of T3 and fT3.

Another possible pathogenetic factor in hypothyroidism in thalassemic patients may be damage by free radicals [7–9]. Chronic hypoxia and an overload of free iron should favour the formation of intermediate products of aerobic metabolism, with an excess of free radicals which are toxic by way of lipid peroxidation and subsequent cellular death. This fact should explain the positive action of iron-chelation therapy in reducing noxious effects of a large amount of free radicals. Therefore, we must pay attention to the role of free radicals in the evaluation of endocrine tissue damage in the thalassemic patient, stressing the importance of proper iron-chelation therapy with desferrioxamine, and that the use of anti-oxidative substances, "scavengers" that are able to reduce the toxic action of free radicals, in the present therapeutic protocols should be taken into consideration.

References

1. Castriota Scanndemberg A, Fenozzi F, Butturini A, Izzi G, Zavota L, Casa F, Giovanneli G (1990) Lo studio del sovraccarico di ferro in soggetti talassemici mediante risonanza magnetica nuclear. Riv Ital Pediatr 16: 294–299
2. De Sanctis V et al. (1990) Prevalence of endocrine complications in patients with beta-thalassemia major. J Endocrinol Invest 13 [Suppl 3]: 114
3. Chatziliami A, Mengreli C, Katsantoni A et al. (1991) Thyroid function in thalassemia. Congres International sur les Maladies Génétique de l'Hémoglobine, Nov, Nice-Acropolis
4. Martino E, Lai E, Balzano S et al. (1991) Thyroid function in thalassemia. Congres International sur les Maladies Génétique de l'Hémoglobine, Nov, Nice-Acropolis
5. Magro S, Puzzonia P, Consarino C et al. (1990) Hypothyroidism in patients with thalassemic syndromes. Acta Haematol (Basel) 84: 72–76
6. Martino E, Lai E, Balzano S, Murtas ML, Figus A (1990) Thyroid function in thalassemia. J Endocrinol Invest 13 [Suppl 3]: 99
7. Halliwell B (1989) Protection against tissue damage in vivo by desferrioxamine: what is its mechanism of action? Free Radic Biol Med 7: 645–651
8. Bompiani GD, Galluzzo A (1990) Radicali liberi in fisiologia e patologia. Minerva Medica, Torino
9. Bacon B, Britton R (1990) The pathology of hepatic iron overload: a free radical-mediated process? Hepatology 2: 127–137

Pituitary-Thyroid Function in Children with β-Thalassemia major*

H. E. Tutar, G. Öcal, N. Akar, and A. Arcasoy

Long-term survival of patients with thalassemia major has been improved by regular transfusion and chelation therapy [1]. However, multiple endocrine disturbances, including thyroid dysfunction, attributed to the chronic transfusional iron overload and causing morbidity and mortality in thalassemic patients are still a major problem [2, 3]. The purpose of the present study was to determine the incidence of pituitary-thyroid dysfunction and its relationship to various clinical and laboratory measurements in thalassemic patients.

Patients and Methods

The study was carried out in the Pediatric Hematology and Endocrinology Departments of Ankara University. Twenty-one (12 male, nine female) transfusion-dependent patients with β-thalassemia major were enrolled; diagnosis was based on clinical, hematological and genetic criteria. Their mean age was 15.15 ± 4.29 years with a range of $10-22.5$ years. All the patients had been multitransfused since early childhood according to a monthly regimen aiming at maintaining pretransfusional hemoglobin levels above $8-9$ g/dl. The study group had regular subcutaneous desferrioxamine infusions ($40-60$ mg/kg, $4-5$ days a week) for the past 5 years.

The pituitary-thyroid axis was evaluated under basal conditions of T4, T3, FT4, FT3, and TSH, and as TSH response to administration of 200 μg i. v. TRH. Blood samples were taken for determination of TSH 20 min before and 30 and 60 min after TRH injection. Nineteen healthy subjects (ten male, nine female) aged $10-26$ years (mean 13.88 ± 3.35) served as controls. Blood samples were taken from all controls for analysis of basal T4, T3, FT4, FT3 and TSH. Fourteen of these were randomly selected for a TRH stimulation test. Informed consent was obtained from all patients and controls or their parents. A commercial radioimmunoassay was used to determine serum concentrations of thyroid hormones and TSH.

A concentration of TSH above the upper range of the values of the controls was accepted as increased (controls: TSH range $0.93-4.20$ μIU/ml; mean = 2.08 ± 0.76), and a concentration of FT4 < 2 SD of the mean control value was defined as decreased (controls: FT4 range $10.9-25.0$ pmol/l; mean = 17.54 ± 4.57).

* This study was supported in part by the Ankara University Research Council and the Ankara Thalassemia Society.

S. Andò et al. (Eds.)
Endocrine Disorders in Thalassemia
© Springer-Verlag Berlin Heidelberg 1995

In addition, a peak value of TSH after TRH injection and a maximal increase above basal value ($\triangle$ TSH) was determined for each patient and control.

Functional status of the pituitary-thyroid axis was defined as normal (normal TSH and FT4), subclinical primary hypothyroidism (HT), (normal basal TSH and FT4; increased TSH response after TRH stimulation), compensated primary HT (increased TSH and normal FT4), uncompensated primary HT (increased TSH and decreased FT4), and secondary HT (normal or low basal TSH and FT4; blunted TSH response to TRH).

The heigth and bone age were determined for all patients. Data were also obtained on mean transfusion requirement, total transfusion time, mean hemoglobin, serum transaminase (ALT, AST) activities, and ferritin values.

Statistical anaylses were performed using Student's t-test; $p < 0.05$ was considered significant.

Results

Pituitary-thyroid dysfunction was found in nine (42.8 %) of the 21 patients. Five of them had subclinical primary HT, two compensated primary HT, one uncompensated primary HT, and one secondary HT. Only 12 patients (57.2 %) were euthyroid. One patient in the euthyroid group had a pattern of hormone levels characteristic of the low T3 syndrome (TSH, T4, FT4 concentrations were normal; T3 and FT3 levels were low). None of the patients with thyroid dysfunction had clinical symptoms of HT.

Patients were divided into two groups according to their thyroid function; patients with thyroid dysfunction, including the patient who had low T3 syndrome (group 1, $n = 10$), and patients with normal thyroid function (group 2, $n = 11$).

Patients with thalassemia major had decreased values of T3, T4 and FT4 as compared with the controls. The mean basal, peak, and $\triangle$ TSH values were high in the thalassemic patients, but there was no statistical difference. Group 2 patients also had decreased FT4 values as compared with the control group; however, peak TSH and $\triangle$ TSH values were significantly low (Table 1).

The mean age of group-1 patients was not statistically different from that of patients in group 2, but severe forms of HT (compensated, uncompensated primary, and secondary HT) were observed only in patients above 15 years old.

There was no statistically significant correlation between impairment of thyroid function and serum ferritin levels, mean transfusion requirement, mean hemoglobin value, and transaminase activity. Although the height and bone age retardation was very prominent in thalassemic patients, there was no difference between the subgroups.

Discussion

Pituitary-thyroid axis and thyroid gland functions in thalassemia major have been reported in a wide spectrum, ranging from normal [2, 4], to subclinical HT [5, 6],

Table 1. Serum thyroid hormones (total and free) and basal, peak, and △ TSH in controls and thalassemic patients

		T3 (μg/ml)	T4 (μg/dl)	FT3 (pmol/l)	FT4 (pmol/l)
A	Control subjects (n = 19)	1.46 ± 0.47	9.85 ± 1.99	6.39 ± 1.62	17.54 ± 4.57
B	All thalassemic patients (n = 21)	1.08 ± 0.33	7.88 ± 1.98	5.49 ± 1.98	12.57 ± 3.11
C	Group 1 (n = 10)	0.96 ± 0.32	6.88 ± 2.29	4.43 ± 1.98	11.23 ± 3.15
D	Group 2 (n = 11)	1.18 ± 0.32	8.79 ± 1.12	6.45 ± 1.47	13.80 ± 2.64
p-Values					
-A vs B		< 0.01	< 0.01	n.s.	< 0.001
-A vs C		< 0.01	< 0.001	< 0.01	< 0.001
-A vs D		n.s.	n.s.	n.s.	< 0.05
		TSH basal (μIU/ml)	TSH peak (μIU/ml)	△ TSH (μIU/ml)	
A	Control subjects (n = 14)	2.26 ± 0.75	15.67 ± 2.72	13.40 ± 2.51	
B	All thalassemic patients (n = 21)	4.49 ± 6.01	21.59 ± 20.42	17.10 ± 14.98	
C	Group 1 (n = 10)	7.22 ± 8.00	31.45 ± 26.77	24.23 ± 19.69	
D	Group 2 (n = 11)	2.00 ± 0.61	12.63 ± 1.93	10.62 ± 1.83	
p-Values					
-A vs B		n.s.	n.s.	n.s.	
-A vs C		< 0.05	< 0.05	< 0.05	
-A vs D		n.s.	< 0.01	< 0.01	

to compensated and uncompensated HT [7, 8]. In addition to primary HT, low T3 syndrome has also been reported in patients with β-thalassemia major [8]. Our data showed a high incidence of HT in our thalassemic patients, predominantly in the subclinical form and recognized only with a TRH stimulation test.

The present study documented the existence of both thyroid and pituitary insufficiency in our thalassemic patients. Thyroid insufficiency is clearly evident from the low FT4 and the raised serum TSH levels. However, in patients with normal thyroid fuctions (group 2) who had significantly low mean FT4, in contrast to expectations, peak and △ TSH values in the TRH test were significantly low. These data indicated that although primary thyroid failure was the predominant pathology, relative pituitary insufficiency for TSH also seems to be a probable contributing factor. These results are in accordance with the data of Livadas et al. [9].

We were not able to demonstrate a correlation between pituitary-thyroid axis impairment and iron overload, expressed as serum ferritin levels. However, previous longitudinal studies indicated that iron overload was the main contributing factor to pituitary-thyroid insufficiency [6, 8, 10].

In conclusion, our study emphasizes the importance of early evaluation of the pituitary-thyroid axis in thalassemic patients by simultaneous measurement of basal thyroid hormones and TSH response to TRH because of the high incidence of subclinical HT. If patients are diagnosed in the subclinical period, chelation therapy should be intensified to prevent progressive damage to the thyroid gland and pituitary.

References

1. Zurlo MG, De Stefano P, Borgna-Pignatti C, Di Palma A, Piga A, Melevendi C, Di Gregorio F, Burattini MG, Terzoli S (1989) Survival and causes of death in thalassaemia major. Lancet 1: 27–29
2. Costin G, Kogut MD, Hyman C, Ortega JA (1979) Endocrine abnormalities in thalassemia major. Am J Dis Child 133: 497–502
3. De Sanctis V, Vullo C, Katz M, Wonke B, Hoffbrand VA, Di Palma A, Bagni B (1989) Endocrine complications in thalassemia major. Prog Clin Biol Res 309: 77–83
4. De Luca F, Melluso R, Sobbrio G, Canfora G, Trimarchi F (1980) Thyroid function in thalassemia major. Arch Dis Child 55: 389–392
5. Masala A, Meloni T, Gallisai D, Alagna S, Rovasio PP, Rassu S, Milia AF (1984) Endocrine functioning in multitransfused prepubertal patients with homozygous β-thalassemia. J Clin Endocrinol Metab 58: 667–670
6. De Sanctis V, D'Ascola G, Tanas R, Vullo C, Bagni B (1985) Preclinical hypothyroidism in patients with β-thalassemia major. In: Sirchia G, Zanella A (eds) Thalassemia today: the Mediterranean experience. CTOMPM, Milan, pp 271–274
7. Magro S, Puzzonia P, Consarino C, Galati MC, Morgione S, Porcelli D, Grimaldi S, Tancré D, Arcuri V, De Sanctis V, Alberti A (1990) Hypothyroidism in patients with thalassemia syndromes. Acta Haematol (Basel) 84: 72–76
8. Sabato AR, De Sanctis V, Atti G, Capra L, Bagni B, Vullo C (1983) Primary hypothyroidism and the low T3 syndrome in thalassaemia major. Arch Dis Child 58: 120–127
9. Livadas DP, Sofroniadou K, Souvatzoglou A, Boukis M, Siafaka L, Koutras DA (1984) Pituitary and thyroid insufficiency in thalassaemic haemosiderosis. Clin Endocrinol 20: 435–443
10. Cavallo L, Licci D, Acquafredda A, Marranzini M, Beccasio R, Scardino ML, Altomare M, Mastro F, Sisto L, Schettini F (1984) Endocrine involvement in children with β-thalassemia major. Transverse and longitudinal studies. I. Pituitary-thyroidal axis function and its correlation with serum ferritin levels. Acta Endocrinol (Copenh) 107: 49–53

Thyroid Function in Thalassemia major

A. Filosa, S. Di Maio, A. Saviano, and S. Aponte

Introduction

Hypothyroidism is one of the most frequent endocrinological complications in thalassemic patients [1]. Lack or delay of puberty [2–4], hypoparathyroidism [5], and insulin-dependent diabetes mellitus [6] are concomitant endocrine abnormalities in such patients. It is reported in the literature that these complications are due to iron over load at the hypothalamic and/or pituitary level and/or at the glandular level [7–9]. Nevertheless, the cause of hypothyroidism in thalassemic patients is unclear still in fact, the results presented in the literature show a broad spectrum of possible alterations [6, 9].

We evaluated the natural history of hypothyroidism in thalassemic patients by analyzing at the onset of the study their TSH response to a TRH test and the peripheral thyroid hormones and during 3 years of follow-up monitoring only peripheral thyroid hormones.

Materials and Methods

Fifty thalassemic patients, aged 10.2–21.3 years (23 male, 27 female) were studied. All patients were currently being treated in the 29th Pediatrics Division of Cardarelli Hospital in Naples.

All patients had been on a regular transfusion program since 1980, every 2–3 weeks, in order to keep their pretransfusional hemoglobin value greater than 10.5 g/dl; nineteen of the patients had received, during the first years of life (mean 2.2 ± 0.7), blood transfusions in order to maintain the Hb value greater than 8 g/dl. Each patient received 40–50 mg/kg/day of deferoxamine by subcutaneous infusion.

A TRH test (5 µg/kg as a bolus i. v.) made possible the determination of the intrinsic TSH secretory reserve. Blood samples were taken for determination of TSH 10 and 0 min before and 10, 20, 30, 45, 60 90, 120 and 180 min after injection. Normal values for our laboratory were: basal TSH 5 ± 1.2 µU/ml $(M \pm SD)$; FT4 0.78 pmol/l as lower limit of the normal value.

Every 3 months serum levels of thyroxine (T4), triodo thyronine (T3), free T4 (FT4), free T3 (FT3), reverse T3 (rT3), thyroid-stimulating hormone (TSH, thyroxine-binding globulin (TBG), thyroglobulin (Tg), and cytoplasm-specific antibodies

S. Andò et al. (Eds.)
Endocrine Disorders in Thalassemia
© Springer-Verlag Berlin Heidelberg 1995

AbTg were determined by radioimmunoassay. All tests were performed 2 days before or 15 days after a transfusion.

According to the criteria of Faglia et al. [10] (Table 1), based on TSH response to TRH and on characteristics of the curve, patients were divided into four groups. Twenty healthy subjects, mean age 15.34 ± 3.07 years (11 male, 9 female), were studied as controls.

Statistical analysis was performed using Student's t-test in order to evaluate differences between the groups of patients, statistically significant at $p < 0.05$. We utilized linear regression to analyze data.

Results

We characterized four groups of patients:

Group 1: euthyroid patients, mean age 13.45 years (13 M, 15 F), showed normal basal TSH, normal FT4, normal $\triangle$ TSH, and a prolonged curve (four patients had a normal curve).

Group 2: 12 patients, mean age 15.83 years, (5 M, 7 F), showed normal basal TSH, normal FT4, exaggerated $\triangle$ TSH, and a prolonged curve (two patients had a normal curve).

Group 3: 6 patients, mean age 16.62 years, (3 M, 3 F), showed compensated hypothyroidism: increased basal TSH, normal FT4, exaggerated $\triangle$ TSH, prolonged curve.

Group 4: 4 patients, mean age 16.87 years (2 M, 2 F), showed uncompensated hypothyroidism: increased basal TSH, low FT4, exaggerated $\triangle$ TSH, and prolonged curve.

Controls: 20 patients showed normal basal TSH, normal FT4, normal $\triangle$ TSH, and a normal curve.

Table 2 shows laboratory data of the patients and controls. No significant statistical correlation was found between FT4 values, ferritin levels before and during the study, age at first transfusion, pretransfusional Hb level, and requirements of packed red blood cells (ml/kg/year) in each group of patients ($p > 0.05$). Table 3 shows clinical characteristics of the four groups of patients. A significant statistical difference was found in ferritin levels between group 4 and groups 1, 2, and 3 ($p < 0.001$).

In group 2, a negative correlation was found between the age of the patients and FT4 values ($r = -0.72$). A significant statistical difference in TSH values at time 180 was found between group 1 and groups 2, 3, and 4 ($p < 0.01$), while no difference was found between group 1 and controls ($p > 0.05$). No significant statistical difference in FT4, FT3, TSH and HPRL peak was found between male and female patients in the same group ($p > 0.05$).

After 3 years of follow-up, five patients of group 2 showed an evolution to compensated hypothyroidism.

Of the 19 older patients who had been receiving a transfusion regimen for some years with pretransfusional hemoglobin level greater than 8 g/dl five patients (17%) were in group 1, seven patients (41%) in group 2, three patients (50%) in

Table 1. Criteria of Faglia et al. for evaluating TSH response to TRH [10]

Response	Net increase △ TSH	Response	Characteristic of the curve
Normal	M 4.5–15 F 6–30	Normal	TSH value at time 60 < TSH value at time 20 TSH value 60 m' after peak smaller than 40 % of the TSH peak value
Imparied	M 1–4.5 F 1–6	Delayed	TSH value at time 60 > TSH value at time 20
Exaggerated	M > 15 F > 30	Prolonged	TSH value 60 m' after peak greater than 40 % of the TSH peak value

Table 2. Levels of FT4, FT3, TSH, △ TSH, peak TSH, peak HPRL, in the four groups and controls (C)

Group	FT3 pmol/l	FT4 pmol/l	TSH µU/ml	△ TSH		Peak TSH		Peak HPRL
1	4.35 ± 1.17	1.204 ± 0.25	1.83 ± 0.80	(13M) (15F)	12.33 ± 2.57 16.26 ± 6.19	(13M) (15F)	14.20 ± 3.56 17.92 ± 5.67	35.85 ± 15.1
2	3.30 ± 0.81	1.216 ± 0.29	1.85 ± 0.81	(5M) (7F)	23.62 ± 6.97 38.34 ± 8.32	(5M) (7F)	25.90 ± 5.98 41.52 ± 9.87	36.95 ± 15.1
3	3.84 ± 0.58	1.245 ± 0.38	8.06 ± 1.28	(3M) (3F)	50.03 ± 1.78 47.90 ± 2.59	(3M) (3M)	59.36 ± 2.01 56.73 ± 3.04	31.20 ± 10.2
4	3.77 ± 1.19	0.527 ± 0.22	23.40 ± 11.5	(2M) (2F)	72.40 ± 3.60 58.05 ± 10.8	(2M) (2F)	99.20 ± 9.92 80.40 ± 9.56	33.60 ± 11.2
C	5.21 ± 0.87	1.184 ± 0.25	3.34 ± 1.24	(11M) (9F)	14.65 ± 3.01 17.43 ± 5.57	(11M) (9F)	16.65 ± 2.67 19.43 ± 4.21	34.78 ± 12.7

Table 3. Clinical characteristics of the four patient groups

Group	Mean age (years)	Age at diagnosis (months)	Ferritin (a) ng/ml	Ferritin (b) ng/ml	Blood requirement (ml/kg/year)
1	13.45 ± 2.91	13.26 ± 12.67	2353 ± 1089	2275 ± 899	175 ± 20
2	15.83 ± 2.31	11.08 ± 7.65	2900 ± 1137	3166 ± 1867	168 ± 15
3	16.62 ± 2.51	6.52 ± 3.53	2116 ± 702	2066 ± 445	178 ± 18
4	16.87 ± 1.94	10.58 ± 5.12	3900 ± 1321	4200 ± 2925	173 ± 16

group 3, and four (100%) in group 4. No correlation was found between age at diagnosis, duration of such a transfusion regimen, and degree of hypothyroidism.

All patients of groups 3 and 4 were affected by hypogonadotropic hypogonadism. No patient was affected by insulin-dependent diabetes mellitus.

Discussion

Overt hypothyroidism represents the final clinical picture of thyroid dysfunction. A temporal evolution, ranging from normal to impaired, is observed in thalassemic patients. This evolution can occur over a variable length of time. The intermediate steps are represented by a broad spectrum of clinical pictures, the causes of which are not satisfactorily explained. Our study showed that at the onset of thyroid complications, all patients had slight damage, both at the glandular level and at the hypothalamic/pituitary level.

In order to assess progressive severity of thyroid disorder, besides thyroid hormone serum levels, serum TSH response to TRH was subdivided into four categories, according to kagnitude of the increase of serum TSH after TRH administration and the pattern of the response curve.

All patients showed a prolonged curve after the TRH test and some of them showed also an exaggerated curve. After 3 years of follow-up, five patients with an exaggerated TSH response to TRH showed an evolution to compensated hypothyroidism. No correlation was found between duration of the transfusion regimen at a low hemoglobin level (7–8 g/dl) and degree of hypothyroidism; furthermore, no correlation was found between thyroid dysfunction and age, FT4, FT3, basal TSH, or HPRL peak. Although a significant statistical difference was found in ferritin levels between group 4 and the other groups, a high serum ferritin level may not reflect the body's iron status, as for example, in patients with chronic hepatitis. On the contrary, patients with low ferritin levels were affected by hypothyroidism. It is important to note that all patients of groups 3 and 4 had concomitant hypogonadtropic hypogonadism. In the absence of a characterized pathological mechanism, some authors reported that damage could be due to hypoxia secondary to anemia in the first years of life [12], that iron absorbed at the intesinal level could produce irreversible tissue damage [13, 14], or, finally, that thyroid gland was more sensible than the hypothalamic-hypophyseal axis to iron overload. None of these causes was recognized in our patients. In conclusion, we suppose that hypothyroidism is a dynamic disease; for this reason, each phase of thyroid disease could be due to a different, still unknown pathological mechanism.

References

1. Magro S et al. (1990) Hypothyroidism in patients with thalassemia syndromes. Acta Hematol Basel 84: 72–76
2. Borgna-Pignatti C, De Stefano P, Zonta MS et al. (1985) Growth and sexual maturation in thalassemia major. J Pediatr 106: 150–155

3. Borgna-Pignatti C (1966) Growth and puberty in thalassemia major. An iterim report. In: Sirchia G, Zanella A, (eds) Milan, Thalassemia today. pp 90–95
4. Kletzky OA, Costin G, Marrs RP et al. (1979) Gonadotropin insufficiency in patients with thalassemia major. J Clin Endocrinol Metab 48: 901–905
5. Clayton BE, Fairmy A, Flynn DM et al. (1976) Parathyroid function in infants and children. In: Bickel H, Ster J (eds) Inborn errors of calcium and bone metabolism. Medical and Technical Publishing, Lancaster
6. Modell B, Berdonkas V (1984) The clinical approach to thalassemia. Grune and Stratton, New York, pp 196–198
7. Costin G, Kogut MD, Hyman CB et al. (1979) Endocrine abnormalities in thalassemia major. Am J Dis Child 133: 497–502
8. Canale VC, Steinherz P, New NZ, Erlandson M (1966) Endocrine function in thalassemia major. Ann NY Acad Sci 232: 333–345
9. McIntosh N (1976) Endocrinopathy in thalassemia major. Arch Dis Child 51: 195–201
10. Faglia G et al. (1979) Thyrotropin secretion in patients with central hypothyroidism: evidence for reduced biological activity of immunoreactive thyrotropin. J Clin Endocrinol Metab 48: 989–999
11. Sabato AR, De Sanctis V, Atti G et al. (1983) Primary hypothyroidism and the low T3 syndrome in thalassemia major. Arch Dis Child 58: 120–127
12. Correra A, Graziano JH, Seaman C et al. (1984) Inappropriately low red cell 2, 3-diphosphoglycerate and p50 in transfused β-thalassemia. Blood 63: 803–806
13. Cavill I, Ricketss C, Jacobs A et al. (1978) Erythropoiesis and the effect of transfusion in homozygous betathalassemia. N Engl J Med 298: 776–780
14. Erlandson ME, Walden B, Stern G et al. (1962) Studies on congenital haemolytic syndromes. IV. Gastrointestinal absorption of iron. Blood 19: 359–378

Pituitary-Gonadal Response to Short-term Pulsatile Luteinizing Hormone-Releasing Hormone Administration in Young Thalassemic Patients

M. Giusti, S. Valenti, P. G. Mori, R. Guido, C. Micalizzi, F. Perfumo, and G. Giordano

Introduction

Delayed puberty is one of the most common endocrine problems in severe thalassemia [1]. Because of its clinical and psychological manifestations it remains a serious problem, especially for male patients. Impaired secretion of both luteinizing hormone (LH) and follicle-stimulation hormone after LH-releasing hormone (LHRH) and, to a lesser extent, a decrease in sex-steroid secretion have been ascribed to pituitary and/or testicular damage by chronic iron overload [2]. However, because pubertal changes are linked to an increase in hypothalamic LHRH activity [3], a defect in the central operator of pubertal activation in thalassemia can also be hypothesized. On the other hand, hypothalamic dysfunction has been suggested in the early stage of genetic hemochromatosis [4]. An impairment in LHRH discharge has been recently described in uremic boys, in whom delayed puberty is a common finding [5], and short-term pulsatile LHRH administration seems to restore normal pituitary-gonadal secretion in uremic boys with delayed puberty [5]. We studied the effect of short-term pulsatile LHRH administration in a group of thalassemic patients with delayed or disordered puberty in order to evaluate the degree of hypothalamic involvement.

Material and Methods

The study was conducted in five thalassemic (age range 15–19 years) and five uremic (14–15 years) boys with delayed puberty. As a control group seven boys (14–17 years) with constitutional delayed puberty were studied. Thalassemic boys were on a hypertransfusion protocol and received desferrioxamine. Except for one (case 5: age 19 years, TV 20 ml, Ph 4) who had been treated with exogenous gonadotropins, all thalassemics showed 2–6 ml in testicular volume (TV) and a score of 1–2 according to Tanner's criteria in pubertal hair (Ph). Uremics (TV 2–4 ml, Ph 1–2) were receiving conservative treatment. Controls showed 3–8 ml in TV and 1–2 score in Ph. Pulsatile LHRH (150 ng/kg body wt. sc every 120 min) delivered by means of a protable pump (Zyklomat, Ferring) was administered to each boy for 7 days. On day 0 and day 7 multiple blood samples (every 15 min for 240 min) were collected. On day 7 each pulse of exogenous LHRH was identified and specimens were collected at the actual moment of drug delivery. On

S. Andò et al. (Eds.)
Endocrine Disorders in Thalassemia
© Springer-Verlag Berlin Heidelberg 1995

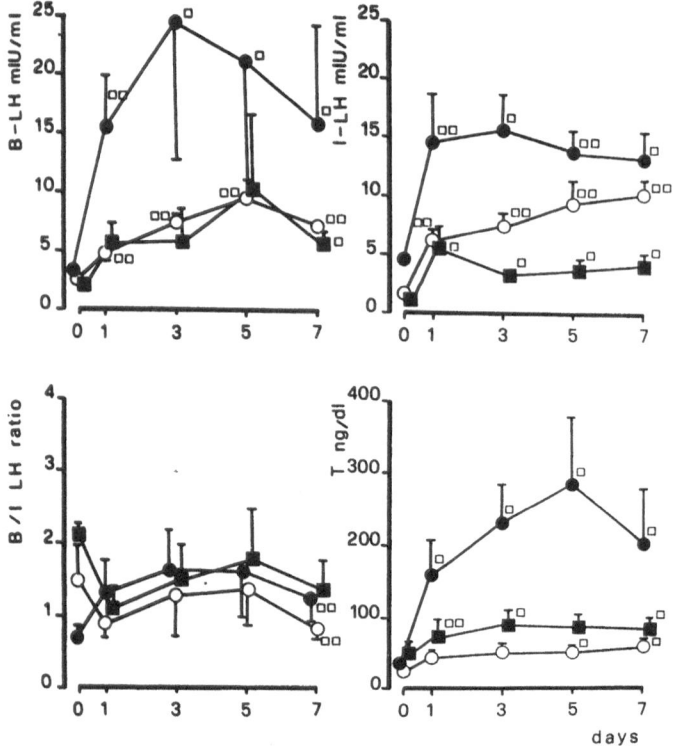

Fig. 1. Behavior of B–LH, I–LH, B/I LH ratio, and T in thalassemic (■—■) uremic (●—●), and control (○—○) subjects from day 0 to day 7 during LHRH administration (□ $p < 0.05$, □□ $p < 0.01$ vs day 0)

days 1, 3, and 5 basal samples were collected 60 min after LHRH delivery. Immunological LH (I–LH) and testosterone (T) were assayed by RIA. Biological LH (B–LH) was assayed according to the Dufau method [6] with minor modifications [5]. The results are presented as the mean ± SE. Statistical analysis among groups was performed on LOG-transformed data by means of ANOVA for randomized blocks at specific time intervals. Further analysis was performed by means of Student's t-test. Within each group of subjects changes from day 0 were evaluated by means of the paired t-test.

Results

Hormonal data collected on day 0 are reported in Fig. 1. I–LH was significantly different among groups ($p < 0.01$). In uremics I–LH (4.5 ± 0.9 mIU/ml) and thalassemic patients (1.7 ± 0.3 mIU/ml). No differences in B–LH, T, and the B/I LH ratio were noted on day 0 (Fig. 1). The pituitary-gonadal response to short-term LHRH administration was varied widely among thalassemic subjects (Fig. 2). A significant I–LH, B–LH, and T increase from day 0 to day 7 was found in each

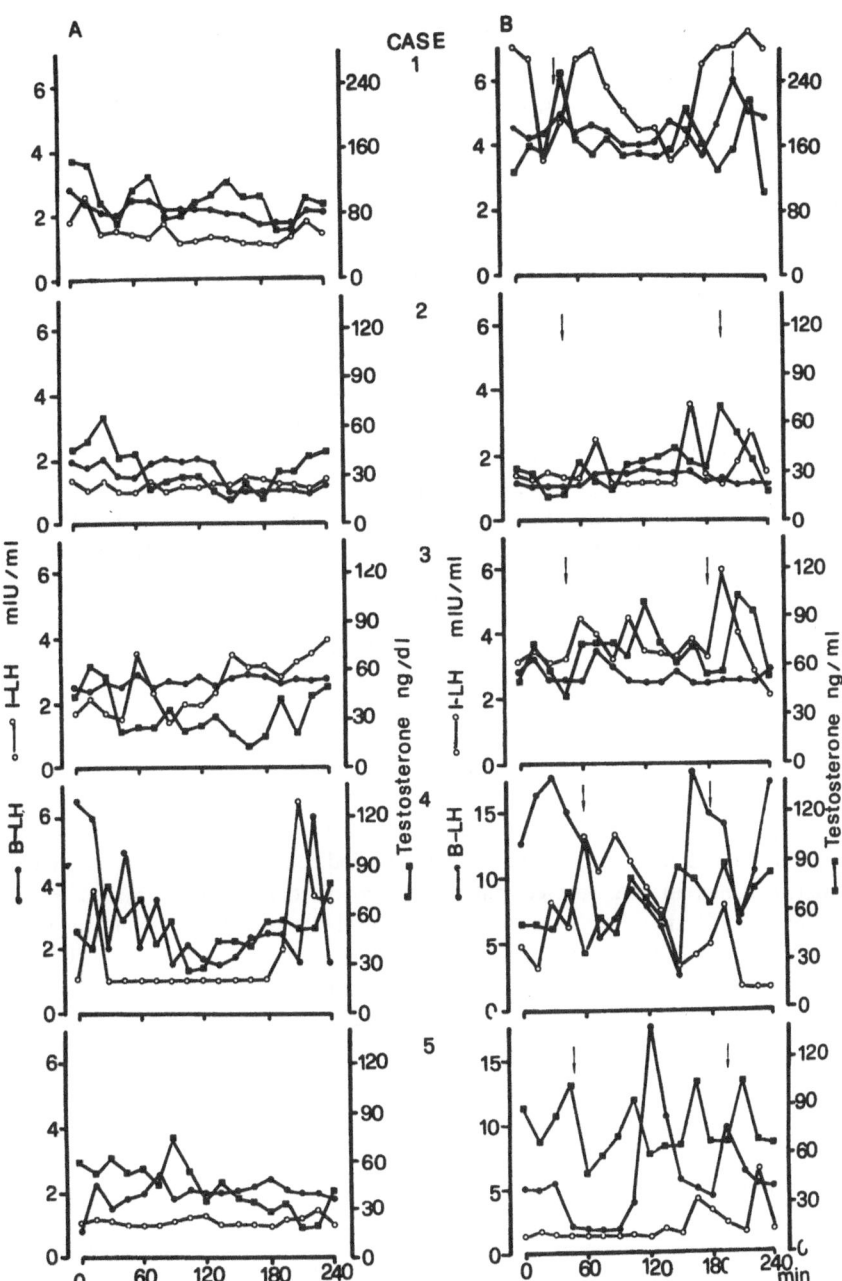

Fig. 2A, B. Individual B–LH, I–LH, and T on day 0 *(panel A)* and day 7 *(panel B)* in the thalasse-mic patients studied. *Arrows* in panel B represent the moment of LHRH infusion

group of subjects (Fig. 1). On day 7 I–LH was significantly lower in thalassemic boys (4.1 ± 1.3 mIU/ml) than in uremics (12.2 ± 2.6 mIU/ml; $p < 0.05$) and controls (10.8 ± 1.7 mIU/ml; $p < 0.05$). No significant differences in B–LH, B/I LH, and T were found among groups on day 7 (Fig. 1).

Discussion

Delayed on disordered puberty is a common feature in uremia [8] and severe thalassemia [1]. Both neuroendocrine (CNS, hypothalamus) [5,8] and peripheral (pituitary, gonads) [2, 9, 10] alterations due to these chronic illnesses have been hypothesized to explain the impairment in the pituitary-gonadal axis. LH bioactivity is regarded as a highly sensitive indicator of endogenous LHRH secretion [11]. The increase of the low B–LH levels after short-term pulsatile LHRH treatment could be regarded as an index of neuroendocrine involvement in both diseases.

Our data document the fact that impaired activity of the pituitary-gonadal axis can be reversed in thalassemic boys, as already shown in uremic and nonuremic boys with delayed puberty (5, present study) after 7 days of pulsatile LHRH administration. A disturbed endogenous LHRH discharge could be hypothesized in uremia [5, 12] and has already been suggested in boys with constitutional delayed puberty [11]. In a previous study, Wang et al. [2] were unable to observe in three thalassemic (1 male, 2 female) subjects aged 17–26 years any change in LH secretion after 6 months of pulsatile LHRH administration. In contrast, our study documents qualitative (B–LH) more than quantitative (I–LH) changes in LH secretion in thalassemic boys during short-term LHRH treatment. Furthermore, the increase in T levels, which can be regarded as an in vivo bioassay, underlines the intact potential of Leydig's cells in both thalassemic and uremic patients. The behavior of LH and T on pulsatile LHRH administration could be indicative of an involvement of the hypothalamus in the delayed puberty of young thalassemic subjects. Recently similar conclusions were reached regarding both preclinical hypogonadism in genetic hemocrohromatosis, where the secretion capacity of LH is intact [4], and young thalassemic women, in whom amenorrhea is probably linked at first to abnormalities in spontaneous LH pulsatility [13].

References

1. Borgna-Pignatti C, De Stefano P, Zonta L, Vullo C, De Sanctis V, Melevendi C, Naselli A, Masera G, Terzoli S, Gabutti V, Piga A (1985) Growth and sexual maturation in thalassemia major. J Pediatr 106: 150–155
2. Wang C, Tso SC, Todd D (1989) Hypogonadotropic hypogonadsism in severe B-thalassemia: effect of chelation and pulsatile gonadotropin-releasing hormone therapy. J Clin Endocrinol Metab 68: 511–516
3. Ducharme JR (1989) Normal puberty: clinical manifestations and their endocrine control. In: Collu R, Ducharme JR, Guyda HJ (eds) Pediatric endocrinology. Raven, New York, pp 307–330

4. Piperno A, Rivolta MR, D'Alba R, Fargio S, Rovelli F, Ghezzi A, Micheli M, Fiorelli G (1992) Preclinical hypogonadism in genetic hemochromatosis in the early stage of the disease: evidence of hypothalamic dysfunction. J Endocrinol Invest 15: 423–128

5. Giusti M, Perfumo F, Verrina E, Cavallero D, Piaggio G, Valenti S, Gusmano R, Giordano G (1992) Delayed puberty in uremia: pituitary-gonadal function during short-term pulsatile luteinizing hormone-releasing hormone administration. J Endocrinol Invest 15: 709–717

6. Dufau ML, Pock R, Neubauer A, Catt KJ (1976) In vitro bioassay of LH in human serum: the interstitial cell testosterone (RICT) assay. J Clin Endocrinol Metab 42: 958–969

7. Scharer K, Schaefer F, Trott M, Kassmann K, Gilli G, Gerhard I, Klinga K, Schonberg D, Vecsei P (1989) Pubertal development in children with chronic renal failure. In: Scharer K (ed) Pediatric and adolescent endocrinology. Karger, Basel, pp 151–168

8. Masala A, Meloni T, Gallisai D, Alagna S, Rovasio PP, Rassu S, Milia AF (1984) Endocrine functioning in multitransfused prepubertal patients with homozygous B-thalassemia. J Clin Endocrinol Metab 58: 667–670

9. Balducci R, Toscano V, Finocchi G, Municchi G, Mangiantini A, Boscherini B (1990) Effect of hCG or hCG + FSH treatments in young thalassemic patients with hypogonadotropic hypogonadism. J Endocrinol Invest 13: 1–7

10. Holdsworth S, Atkins RC, De Kretser DM (1977) The pituitary testicular axis in men with chronic renal failure. N Engl J Med 296: 1245–1249

11. Tsatsoulis A, Shalet SM, Robertson WR (1991) Bioactive gonadotrophin secretion in man. Clin Endocrinol (Oxf) 35: 193–206

12. Veldhuis JD, Wilkowski MJ, Zwart AD, Urban RJ, Lizarralde G, Iranmanesh A, Bolton WK (1993) Evidence for attenuation of hypothalamic-releasing hormone (GnRH) impulse strength with preservation of GnRH pulse frequency in men with chronic renal failure. J Clin Endocrinol Metab 76: 648–654

13. Chatterjee R, Katz M, Wonke B, Porter JB (1992) Long-term follow-up of hypothalamic-pituitary axis in patients with secondary amenorrhoea. International Mediterranean Conference on Endocrine Disorders in Thalassemia, May 7–9, Cosenza, p 20

Long-term Gonadotropin Administration to Restore Gonadal Function in Male Thalassemics

R. Fadini, M. R. Rivolta, W. Monguzzi, E. Lanzi,
M. Mignini-Renzini, and A. L. Boneschi

Introduction

A considerable number of patients with β-thalassemia major reach the pubertal age today; regular development of sexual characteristics and a normal reproductive life are important goals for these patients [1]. Absence of pubertal development is seen in 40% of male thalassemics; abnorml sexual maturation is present in 79% [2].

Sex steroids, gonadotropins, and GnRH are therapeutic agents available to induce puberty and fertility in male thalassemics [3, 4]. In this study we evaluated the effectiveness of chronic administration of hCG and FSH to induce and maintain pubertal development and to affect semen parameters in thalassemic patients.

Patients and Methods

Nine male patients with β-thalassemia major were evaluated. All were aged between 13 and 27 years (mean 18.2 ± 4.5 years). Their mean height was 152 ± 14.5 cm. Sexual maturation was assessed according to Tanner's criteria [5]: four patients were prepubertal (T1); two were in early puberty (T2–3), and three were in mid puberty (T4). Cryptorchidism was present in three subjects.

Semen analysis was performed in all patients: aspermia was observed in seven cases, azoospermia in two.

All patients received hCG: the starting dose was 1000 IU i.m. twice weekly. During the treatment period dose adjustments were made based on serum testosterone levels. FSH was added at a starting dose of 500 IU i.m. twice weekly, when Tanner stage 4–5 was achieved.

Patients were reviewed every 3 months. At each visit a complete physical examination, serum testosterone assays, and semen analysis were performed. Treatment duration ranged between 12 and 46 months.

Results

Eight patients required a dose increase of hCG to maximum of 3000 IU i.m. twice weekly. Two patients required an increase of FSH doses to 1000 IU i.m. twice weekly. Eight patients responded to hCG administration with an increase of serum

S. Andò et al. (Eds.)
Endocrine Disorders in Thalassemia
© Springer-Verlag Berlin Heidelberg 1995

testosterone to the normal range within 3 months of treatment. One patient showed no response to hCG therapy.

Full pubertal maturation (Tanner 5) was achieved by four subjects within 9–18 months of therapy. Four patients progressed to late puberty (Tanner 4). Mean height increased from 152.5 ± 14.5 cm to 157 ± 12.5 cm.

All the aspermic patients showed azoospermia during the treatment period. Semen analysis assessed spermatozoa in only two cases after 12 and 30 months respectively: one patient had been aspermic and the other one azoospermic before treatment.

Four patients complained of mild gynecomastia during the first months of therapy; the symptom resolved with continued therapy.

All patients showed good compliance.

Discussion

Intensive transfusion regimens and iron-chelating therapy have improved the life expectancy of patients with thalassemia major [1]. However, abnormal sexual maturation is present in 79% of boys; [2] hypogonadotropic hypogonadism is present in 20–40% of patients who receive adequate chelating therapy and in 70–80% of patients with inadequate therapy.

Therapeutic options in the management of hypogonadotropic hypogonadism are testosterone, GnRH, and gonadotropin. Testosterone has hepatotoxic effects and is controindicated in thalassemic patients with impaired liver function [6].

GnRH administration is not useful in subjects with pituitary abnormality; the pituitary is extremely sensitive to iron toxicity, and even small amounts of iron may produce irreversibile damage [2]. Besides, GnRH is not the treatment of choice for male thalassemics because of its complex administration schedule. hCG administration is effective in inducing secondary sexual characteristics, and the addition of FSH to hCG therapy increases T response to hCG [7, 8]. Our study shows that chronic gonadotropin administration is effective in inducing and maintaining sexual secondary features. This treatment is also able to affect semen characteristics.

Patients showed good compliance to therapy in spite of its duration and the need for parenteral administration. Thus, gonadotropin seems to be the treatment of choice for hypogonadotropic hypogonadism in patients with thalassemia major.

References

1. Pearson HA, Guiliotis DK, Rink L, Wells (1987) Patient age distribution in thalassemia major; changes from 1973 to 1985. Pediatrics 80: 53
2. Borgna Pignatti C, De Stefano P, Zonta L, Vullo C, De Sanctis V, Melevendi C, Maselli A, Masera G, Terzoli S, Gabutti U, Piga A (1985) Growth and sexual maturation in thalassemia major. J Pediatr 106: 150
3. Wilson JD, Griffin JE (1980) The use and misuse of androgens. Metabolism 29: 1278
4. Balducci R, Toscaro V, Casilli D, Maroder M, Sciana F, Boscherini B (1987) Testicular responsiveness following chronic administration of hCG in untreated hypogonadotropic hypogonadism. Horm Metab Res

5. Tanner JM (1962) Growth at adolescence. Blackwell Scientific, Oxford
6. Shephard RJ, Kilinger D, Fried T (1977) Response to sustained use of anabolic steroids. Br J Sports Med 11: 70
7. Matsumoto AM, Paulsen CA, Bremner WJ (1983) Stimulation of sperm production by human luteinizing hormone in gonadotropin-suppressed normal men. J Clin Endocrinol Metab 59: 882
8. Matsumoto AM, Karpas AE, Bremner WJ (1986) Human chorionic gonadotropin administration in normal mean: evidence that follicle-stimulating hormone is necessary for the maintenance of quantitatively normal spermatogenesis in men. J Clin Endocrinol Metab 62: 1184

Pubertal Development in Female Thalassemics

Ö. Gökçen, D. Malyali, E. Kanadikirik, and H. Azizlerli

Although the prognosis of transfusion-dependent thalassemia has improved greatly with more intensive transfusion regimens and chelation therapy, delayed puberty and hypogonadism are still common problems. The purpose of this study was to evaluate and to compare two groups one of which received regular iron chelation therapy and the other irregular iron chelation therapy or none.

Female patients with beta-thalassemia usually suffer from hypogonadotropic hypogonadism associated with amenorrhea, anovulation, and infertility attributed to the deposition of hemosiderin in the pituitary gland as well as in the ovaries.

Today great advances have been achieved in confronting thalassemia. With regular blood transfusions, iron-chelation therapy, and bone marrow transplantation, the survival of patients extending into the fourth and fifth decades of life has been made possible. These patients may naturally marry, have children, and participate actively in social life. For that reason, growth, sexual development, and fertility have become important issues.

We compared the growth rate and sexual maturation of patients who had chelation therapy with patients who did not. All were members of the TADAD (Thalassemia patients-parent association).

Material and Methods

In our study 11 female patients with thalassemia were evaluated and followed up between April 1990 and April 1992. These patients were divided into group A and group B.

Group A included five patients were regularly transfused and iron chelated; their ferritin levels were sufficent. They have spontoneous menstruation or secondary amenorrhea.

Group B included six patients who were irregularly transfused and iron chelated; their ferritin levels were high. They have primary amenorrhea or delayed puberty. For pubertal staging the Tanner-Marshal classification was used. Basal LH, FSH, estradiol, prolactin, testosterone, and DHEA-S levels were determined by RIA. Growth rate and sexual maturation between group A and B were compared. None of them received sex hormo ne replacement before pubertal age.

S. Andò et al. (Eds.)
Endocrine Disorders in Thalassemia
© Springer-Verlag Berlin Heidelberg 1995

Clinical Investigation

All patients in groups A and B were clinically investigated for the following parameters (see Table 1). Pubic and axillary hair, breast development, menarche, measurements of the ovaries and uterus by ultrasonography, and menstrual cycles. All patients in groups A and B had the typical thalassemic appearance. Skin and mucosal membranes were pigmented. In group B, 90% patients were short for their age and rather thin; in group A, the height was not less than the mean for the normal population, but all patients had limited pubic and axillary hair. In five female patients between 13 and 22 years of age in group A, breast development was observed to be normal (Tanner 2–4). These patients had normal estradiol levels and normal menstrual patterns; their average age at menarche was 13.8. Pubic and axillary hair was within normal limits. Ovarian measurements were considered to be normal (average 32.5 x 42 x 21.5 mm). In six female patients between 15 and 24 years of age in group B, little breast development was observed, corresponding to Tanner stage 1–2. These patients had low estradiol levels. Four patients (17, 18, 19, and 24 years old) had been amenorrheic, one patient (15 years old) had been oligomenorrheic, and one patient (26 years old) had delayed puberty. In group pubic and axillary hair were limited (Tanner stage 1–2). These six female patients in group B were found to have hypogonadism. Three patients who had sex hormone replacement between 17 and 19 years of age showed good progress up to Tanner stage 3–4 and started menstruating. On patient (24 years old) was still in Tanner stage 1 at the end of 6 months treatment. One patient refused hormone replacement therapy.

Hormonal Findings

Serum prolactin was normal in both groups. FSH and LH were significantly low in group B. Serum estrodiol in these groups was also found to be low. DHEA-S was low in all of the female subjects.

Table 1. Laboratory and clinical data on 11 patients in groups A and B

Name	Age (years)	Ferritin ( )	Pubertal Studies	FSH (mUL/ml)	LH (pg/ml)	E2	T μ (g/dl)	DHEA-S (ng/dl)	PRL
FC	22	1960	P3 T3	4.7	2.4	41	0.2	650	3.2
AC	21	2100	P3 T4	7.9	7.2	52	0.6	520	10.2
YK	14	1800	P3 T2	6.8	6.4	45.2	0.1	1050	12.4
AY	13	1200	P3 T2	4.9	5.4	41.3	0.2	870	5.3
SC	19	1700	P3 T4	7.2	6.9	51	0.3	620	6.4
Group A									
SS	17	4750	P2 T1	1.4	0.8	9	0.7	450	2.3
AE	15	7300	P1 T1	0.01	0.01	9.2	0.3	670	7.9
NS	18	8400	P1 T2	1.3	1.1	3.9	0.4	540	3.4
EC	24	5200	P2 T1	1.4	1.2	3.4	0.2	650	10.2
EN	26	4300	P2 T2	1.1	0.8	3.8	0.4	670	7.2
BA	19	5900	P1 T1	1.4	1.1	3.1	0.5	910	2.3

E, Estradiol; T, testosterone; DHEA-S, dehydroepiandrosterone; PRL, prolactin

Four female patients in group B received sex hormone replacement therapy for at least 6 months. Three patients showed an increase in sexual characteristics and increased levels of estradiol.

Conclusion

Thalassemia is a very serious disease. It should be treated before the onset of puberty so that children can achieve normal sexual maturation. Patients who fail to enter puberty are believed to be infertile for life. When these patients grow up they feel emotionally deprived; they may become depressed and isolated in the community. Hypertransfusion plus regular, intensive iron chelation and sex hormone replacement may help to establish secondary sex characteristics.

Eleven patients with beta thalassemia were evaluated for growth and sexual development (in group B). Six patients were found to be in Tanner stage 1 or 2. Only five patients had normal rates of pubertal maturation.

We believe that preventing accumulation of iron with intensive chelation therapy in early puberty is the key to normal growth and sexual development. After puberty, this therapy might not be effective enough to reverse the iron-induced damage to the pituitary gland. It is believed that chronic hypoxia and iron deposition in the gonads are the other possible causes. We think that we have to work hard all over the world to understand the real problems and therapy of this disease.

References

1. Anastasi S, Caruso V, Magnano C, Leocata A (1991) The endocrine complications in thalassemia major. Pediatr Med Chir 13(1): p 63–65
2. Ando S, Giaccetto C, Bria M, Tagarelli A, Piro A, Seidita F, Brancati C (1987) Endocrine correlates of adrenal and testicular function with circulating ferritin plasma levels in adult thalassemic patients. Birth Defects 23(5A): 459–468
3. Danesi L, Scacchi M, De Martin M, Dubini A, Massaro P (1992) Evaluation of hypothalamic-pituitary function in patients with thalassemia major. Endocrinol Invest 15(3): 177–186
4. De Sanctis V, Vullo C, Katz M, Wonke B, Tanas R, Bagni B (1988) Gonadal function in patients with beta thalassemia major. Clin Pathol 41(2): 133–137
5. De Sanctis V, Vullo C, Katz M, Wonke B, Hoffbrand VA, Di Palma A (1989) Endocrine complications in thalassemia major. Prog Clin Biol Res 309: 77–83
6. Janssen G, Schuster A, Ranke MB, Gobel U (1991) Combined hypophyseal function test in children with homozygous beta-thalassemia. Klin Padiatr 203: 104–108
7. De Montalembert M, Llados A, Hannedouche T. Girot R (1989) Treatment of posttransfusion iron overload by deferoxamine. Arch Fr Pediatr 46(2): 99–105
8. Mordel N, Birkenfeld A, Goldfarb AN, Rachmilewitz EA (1989) Successful full-term pregnancy in homozygous beta-thalassemia major: case report and review of the literature. Obstet Gynecol 73(52): 837–840
9. Shehadeh N, Hazani A, Rudolf MC, Peleg I, Benderly A, Hochberg Z (1990) Neurosecretory dysfunction of growth hormone secretion in thalassemia major. Acta paediatr Scand 79(8–9): 790–795
10. Vullo C, De Sanctis V, Karz M, Wonke B, Hoffbrand AV (1990) Endocrine abnormalities in thalassemia. Ann NY Acad Sci 612: 293–310

The Pituitary-Thyroid-Gonadal Axis
in Saudi β-Thalassaemia Patients

M. A. F. EL-HAZMI, A. S. WARSY, and I. AL-FAWAZ

Introduction

Beta-thalassaemia major (β-thal. major) patients frequently suffer from endocrine dysfunction, a consequence of the transfusion-related iron overload [1–4]. Deposition of iron in different tissues including the pituitary gland, the thyroid and the gonads has been well documented histologically [2, 5]. The reported endocrine abnormalities include hypoparathyroidism, deficiency of luteinizing hormone (LH), follicle-stimulating hormone (FSH) and thyroid hormone, and impaired function of islet cells of the pancreas [1–4, 6]. Though several studies point to these abnormalities, others present contradictory results and show no variation in some endocrine levels [7]. These discrepancies have been related to ethnic variations and to differences in management strategies. This study was initiated to investigate the pituitary-thyroid-gonadal axis in Saudi β-thalassaemia patients.

Material and Methods

The patients (22 children, aged < 15 years) suffering from β-thal. major were attending the clinics at King Khalid University hospitals, Riyadh for regular transfusion and follow-up. The children were on chelation therapy using desferrioxamine. The control group consisted of 50 normal children attending the outpatient clinics for minor illnesses. Physical examination was carried out and frequency of transfusion was recorded. Blood was drawn and used for the estimation of haematological parameters and red cell indices, using a Coulter Counter ZF. Discriminant factors were calculated. Red cells and buffy coat were removed by centrifugation. Washed red cells, after haemolysis, were used for determination of haemoglobin phenotype on acid and alkaline electrophoresis and for Hb A_2 and Hb F estimations. A fresh blood sample was used to determine the a/non-a globin chain ratio. DNA was extracted from the buffy coat, and the β-thalassaemia mutations were investigated by the Amplification Refractory Mutation System (ARMS) [8]. Plasma was used for the estimation of free triiodothyronine (T3), free thyroxine (T4), follicle-stimulating hormone (FSH), and luteinizing hormone (LH) by a competitive immunoassay technique using the Amerlite Assay kit. Testosterone, growth hormone (GH) and ferritin level were estimated by RIA using kits from Amersham (SAS). Results were fed to computers and analysed using the Statistical Analysis System (SAS).

S. Andò et al. (Eds.)
Endocrine Disorders in Thalassemia
© Springer-Verlag Berlin Heidelberg 1995

Table 1. Haematological parameters (mean ± SD) in β-thal. major patients and control group

Parameter	β-Thal. major	Controls
Hb (g/dl)	9.1 ± 2.2	13.13 ± 0.86
RBC (x10^{12}/l)	2.9 ± 0.7	4.7 ± 0.31
PCV (1/l)	0.25 ± 0.06	0.38 ± 0.02
MCV (fl)	73.7 ± 7.0	87.2 ± 3.3
MCH (pg)	32.0 ± 3.3	31.7 ± 4.5
MCHC (g/dl)	36.0 ± 3.0	38.2 ± 3.3
Hb A$_2$ (%)	3.3 ± 1.8	2.5 ± 0.5
Hb F (%)	7.4 ± 5.8	0.8 ±0.25

Table 2. Ferritin and hormone levels in β-thal. major patients compared with the control group

	β-Thal. major	Control
Ferritin (µg/l)	880 ± 204	83.4 ± 70.3
Hormones:		
fT3 (pmol/l)	5.7 ± 1.8	5.4 ± 0.7
fT4 (pmol/l)	22.7 ± 13.5*	18.6 ± 3.0
FSH (mIU/ml)	1.9 ± 1.45 (F)*	5.8 ± 2.9 (F)
	2.6 ± 1.7 (M)*	4.9 ± 3.3 (M)
LH (mIU/ml)	0.7 ± 0.5 (F)*	13.5 ± 9.6 (F)
	1.4 ± 1.8 (M)*	11.1 ± 7.6 (M)
Testosterone (mmoI/l)	8.3 ± 8.0 (M)	14.2 ± 2.6 (M)
GH (mU/l)	0.5 ± 0.3	1.7 ± 1.3

f, Free; M, male; F, female
* = Difference compared with control group is statistically significant ($p < 0.05$)

Table 3. Frequency of abnormality of hormones in β-thal. major

	β-Thal. major (%)
Deficiency of	
LH	100
FSH	17.5
fT3	18.2
fT4	45

The significance of the difference between the mean of the control group and that of the patients was determined by Student's t-test. $p < 0.05$ was considered statistically significant.

Results

All patients were suffering from β-thalassaemia major as judged from the history of clinical presentation and haematological parameters, red cell indices, a/non-a-globin ratio and results of ARMS. The haematological parameters of the patients compared with the control group are presented in Table 1.

The ferritin and hormone levels in the patients and control group are presented in Table 2. Significant differences were encountered when comparison was made with the control group, the most significant being lower LH and FSH levels. Other hormones such as GH and testosterone were lower, but the differences in the results were not statistically significant. Free T3 (fT3) was similar to the control group but free T4 (fT4) was elevated.

The frequency of deficiency of the fT3, fT4, FSH and LH were calculated and the results are presented in Table 3. Elevation of fT3 and fT4 was encountered in 4.5% and 22.7% of the patients, respectively.

Discussion and Conclusion

The patients investigated in this study were on regular blood transfusion and had received chelation therapy with desferrioxamine regularly. This was ascertained from the ferritin levels, which, though significantly higher than normal, were significantly lower than in patients not given chelation therapy.

From the results of this study, we conclude that β-thal. major patients on regular chelation therapy still have endocrine abnormalities which correlate closely with the extent of their blood transfusion requirement. No correlation was demonstrated between the total ferritin level and the endocrine abnormalities. It appears that once the iron level is elevated in the body it causes an irreversible organ damage. However, this damage may be controlled if chelation therapy is initiated as early as possible, as documented in other studies.

Finally, the pituitary-thyroid-gonadal axis needs to be carefully monitored in children suffering from β-thal. major and hormone replacement therapy may prove to be beneficial.

Acknowledgement. This study was supported partially by grant no. AT-4-074 from King Abdulaziz City for Science and Technology (KACST), Riyadh, and partially by King Saud University, Riyadh.

References

1. Vullo C, De Sanctis V, Katz M, Wonke B et al. (1990) Endocrine abnormalities in thalassaemia. Ann NY Acad Sci 612: 293–310
2. Costin G, Kogut MD, Hyman CB, Ortega JA (1979) Endocrine abnormalities in thalassaemia major. Am J Dis Child 133: 497–502
3. Flynn DM, Fairney A, Jackson D, Clyaton BE (1976) Hormonal changes in thalassaemia major. Arch Dis Child 51: 828–836
4. McIntosh N (1976) Endocrinopathy in thalassaemia major. Arch Dis Child 51: 195–201
5. Fink HE (1964) Transfusion hemochromatosis in Cooley's anemia. Ann NY Acad Sci 119: 680–685
6. De Sanctis V, Zurlo MG, Senesi E, Boffa C, et al. (1988) Insulin-dependent diabetes in thalassaemia. Arch Dis Child 63: 58–62
7. De Luca F, Melluso R, Sobbrio G, et al. (1980) Thyroid function in thalassaemia major. Arch Dis Child 55: 389–392
8. Old JM, Varawalla NY, Weatherall DJ (1990) Rapid detection and prenatal diagnosis of β-thalassaemia: studies in Indian and Cypriot populations in U.K. Lancet 336: 834–837

Insulin-Dependent Diabetes mellitus in a Group of Young People with beta-Thalassemia major

S. Anastasi, V. Caruso, M. Cantone, and C. Magnano

Introduction

The increased survival of thalassemic patients, due largely to the application of new therapeutic methods [1], has brought about a greater incidence of diabetes with thalassemia [2, 3]. The development of diabetes seems to result from the establishment of a pathogenetic mechanism which involves hemosiderosis, liver disease, and insulin resistance, whereas family history and association with other autoimmune pathologies seem to be less evident [4]. The aim of this paper is to evaluate the frequency of diabetes and functional changes in the pancreas thalassemic patients.

Patients and Methods

We studied the pancreatic function of 29 thalassemic major patients (11 male and 18 female) ranging from 10.3 to 27.0 years of age. The patients are part of a group of 76 thalassemic major patients who have been in our care for at least 10 years and have undergone treatment with transfusions; their erythrocyte concentrations and pretransfusion levels of Hb ranged from 8.0 g/dl in 1977 to 10.5 g/dl in 1990. Iron chelating therapy i.m. was begun in 1980; in 1983 it was administered as subcutaneous infusions of deferoxamine (DFX) in 40–60 mg/kg doses 6 days a week. There was an average of 80% compliance to the therapy by the 29 patients studied; most (23) had undergone a splenectomy.

Six patients were found to be suffering from insulin-dependent diabetes mellitus (IDDM) according to the NDDG [5]. Their age at the time of diagnosis was 15–19 years, and the onset of diabetes was preceded in five patients by tenuous clinical signs, ranging from slight weight loss to the progressive development of polyuria and polydipsia. In only one case had ketoacidosis set in.

The metabolic control of diabetes was achieved by means of glycemia and glycosuria tests at home, as well as standard hematochemical tests.

The remaining 23 patients underwent an OGTT. Blood samples were taken every 0, 30, 60, 90, and 120 min to test for glycemia and insulinemia. Periodic checks were carried out on all the patients regarding hepatic, cardiac, thyroid, and gonadal functions, as well as ferritin levels.

S. Andò et al. (Eds.)
Endocrine Disorders in Thalassemia
© Springer-Verlag Berlin Heidelberg 1995

Results

All the diabetic patients received insulin therapy in doses ranging from 0.4 to 1.1 U/kg per day. In only one case was there a family history of IDDM. All the patients presented with other endocrinopathies associated with the diagnosis of diabetes (Table 1). Five of them had hepatic dysfunction and four showed signs of cardiopathy. Ferritin levels were high on average in all cases, except in the patient with familial diabetes.

Seven of 23 patients who underwent OGTT had impaired glucose tolerance. Hyperinsulinism was detected in 11 patients, four of whom showed intolerance and seven a normal glycemic curve response orally.

Other associated endocrinopathies (Table 1) were encountered in eight of the 17 patients with normal responses and in six with impaired glucose metabolism The ferritin serum values varied considerably both in patients with impaired glucose tolerance and in those with a normal response.

All the patients with altered tolerance showed signs of hepatic infection from B or C virus and hepatic weakening with a more or less marked hypertransaminasemia, whereas these signs were present in only 50% of the patients with normal glucose tolerance (Table 2).

Conclusions and Discussion

Patients with thalassemia major have a greater risk of developing IDDM. The accumulation of iron in the hepatic and pancreatic cells and in other endocrine glands could play a fundamental role in the onset of diabetes [2, 6, 7]. We have encounted IDDM in six of 29 patients over the age of 10 years (20.6%). A compari-

Table 1. Other associated endocrine complications in thalassemia major patients

	Normal (n)	Impaired glucose tolerance (n)	Diabetic (n)
Hypothyroidism	1	3	2
Hypoparathyroidism	0	1	2
Hypogonadism	8	6	6

Table 2. Liver function in thalassemia major patients

(%)	Normal n (%)	Impaired glucose tolerance n (%)	Diabetic n
Normal	9 (53)	0	1 (17)
Altered	8 (47)	7 (100)	5 (82)
Hepatitis C	7 (41)	6 (85)	2 (33)
Hyperinsulinism	7 (41)	4 (57)	–

Table 3. Increase in incidence of diabetes among thalassemia major patients over 10 years

	1981	1991
Total no. of patients	67	76
Diabetics	1	6
Impaired glucose tolerance	4	6

son of the incidence of diabetic complications in patients in our care 10 years ago shows a clear increase today, probably due to iron excess brought on by the use of hypertransfusion therapy, beginning in the early 1980s (Table 3) [7].

Our observation of ferritin values, which are, on average, higher in patients with diabetes and glucose intolerance than in those with a normal glucose response, leads us to attribute an important role to hemosiderosis in the development of diabetic complications.

Another important fact to bear in mind is the role of liver disease in determining the development of diabetes in thalassemia [8]. In our experience, five patients with diabetes and all the patients with impaired glucose tolerance showed signs of hepatic infection from B and / or C virus and more or less marked hypertransamina-semia.

The high frequency of other associated endocrinopathies points once again to the presence of iron deposits in the parenchymal cells as a primary factor causing damage to these patient's organs.

As far as the insulin response to glucose is concerned, the observed hyperinsulinism may imply a pathogenetic role of increased peripheral resistance to insulin as a co-factor that would lead to faster breakdown of the b-pancreatic function, combined with an altered hepatic and glucose metabolism as a result of the higher incidence of a liver disease [9, 10]. This experience confirms the role of hemosiderosis and hepatopathy in the onset of diabetes in thalassemia.

References

1. Vullo C, Cao A, Gabutti W, Masera G, Sirchia G (1985) Protocollo per la terapia della β-thalas-semia. Ciba-Geigy, Basel
2. Lassman MN, Genel M, Wise JK, Hendler R, Felig P (1974) Carbohydrate homeostasis and pancreatic islet cell function in thalassemia. Ann Intern Med 80: 65
3. De Sanctis V, Zurlo MG, Senesi E, Boffa C, Cavallo L, Di Gregorio F (1988) Insulin-dependent diabetes in thalassemia. Arch Dis Child 63: 58
4. Lorini R, Cortona L, Martinetti M, Larizza D, Livieri C, D'Annunzio G, Zonta L, Cuccia Belvedere M, Severi F (1989) Studio della eterogeneità clinica, immunologica e genetica del diabete mellito insulino dipendente in età pediatrica. R.I.P. 15: 279 Rivista Italiana di Pediatria
5. National Diabetes Data Group (1979) Classification and diagnosis of diabetes mellitus and other categories of glucose intolerance. Diabetes 28: 1039
6. Anastasi S, Caruso V, Magnano C, Leocata A (1991) Complicanze endocrine nella thalassemia major. Med Surg Pediatr 13: 63
7. Propper RD, Button LN, Nathan DG (1980) New approaches to the transfusion management of thalassemia. Blood 55: 55
8. De Sanctis V, D'Ascola G, Wonke D (1986) The development of diabetes mellitus and chronic disease in long-term chelated thalassemic patients. Postgrad Med J 62: 831

9. Costin G, Cobut MD, Kogut MD, Hyman C, Ortega JA (1977) Carbohydrate metabolism and pancreatic islet-cell function in thalassemia major. Diabetes 26: 230
10. Merkel PA, Simonson DC, Amiel SA, Plewe G, Sherwin RS, Pearson HA, Tamborlane WV (1988) Insulin resistance and hyperinsulinemia in patients with thalassemia major treated by hypertransfusion. N Engl J Med 318: 809

A Transverse and Longitudinal Study of Pancreatic Function and Glucose Tolerance in Thalassemic Patients

L. Cavallo, F. Trentadue, S. Liuzzi, T. Giobbe, R. Leuzzi, V. Sabato, D. De Mattia, and F. Schettini

Polytransfused thalassemia major (Th) patients show a high prevalence (frequently reported > 50%) of impairment of β-pancreatic function (PF) and of overt diabetes mellitus (10–25%). The impairment of liver function, the hyperinsulinemia following insulin resistance, the hyperglucagonemia, the β-pancreas exhaustion, the genetic predisposition, and the increased frequency of viral infections could play a role in the pathogenesis of the PF derangement [1–7]. The prevalence of diabetes mellitus has been reported to be lower in regularly (16%) than in irregularly (23%) iron-chelated Th patients [7]. In this retrospective transverse and longitudinal study we have evaluated the effect of the improvement of chelation and transfusion protocols on the prevalence of PF and of impaired glucose tolerance (GT) in Th patients.

Material and Methods

An oral glucose tolerance test (OGTT) was performed during the past 5 years 1, 2, 3, and 4 times in 38, 34, 7, and 2 Th patients, respectively (interval generally > 1 year). Eleven patients were aged 3–8 years (group A), 42 were aged 8–14 years (group B), and 39 were aged 14–24 years (group C). Two patients changed from group A to group B and seven from group B to group C. All had been regularly transfused with packed red blood cells from the age of 1.1 ± 0.9 years, with a mean pre- and post-transfusional Hb level of 10.3 ± 0.5 and 13.1 ± 1.0 g/dl, respectively. Chelation therapy (desferrioxamine mesylate administered by microinfusion pump: 40–50 mg/kg/day 6 nights/week) was started at 5.0 years (median) and continued for 7.6 years (median; range, 1–12 years). Mean serum ferritin levels were 3286 ± 2019 µg/dl. Twenty-seven patients had been splenectomized at 6.5 years (median; range, 2.1–20.0 years) and two had undergone bone marrow transplantation at the age of 10.2 and 14.1 years, respectively. Patients with congestive heart failure, hypoparathyroidism, hypothyroidism, or GH deficiency and those undergoing endocrine therapy were excluded from the study. The OGTT was performed by administering 40 g/m^2 of glucose (max 75 g) at 9.00 a.m. after an overnight fast. Circulating glucose, insulin (IRI), and C-peptide (C-p) levels were evaluated before and 30, 60, 120, and 180 min after the glucose load. Glycemia was assayed by the glucose-oxidase method and both IRI and C-p by radioimmunological methods using commercial kits (Ares Serono, Italy, and Byc-Sangtec Diagnostica, Germany, respectively). Furthermore, the sum of levels at the different

S. Andò et al. (Eds.)
Endocrine Disorders in Thalassemia
© Springer-Verlag Berlin Heidelberg 1995

times of the OGTT (Σ) was calculated for both blood glucose and IRI and C-p levels. The GT was considered impaired when glycemic values were $> 140 \, mg/dl$ at 60 and/or 120 min, while the insulinemic curve was considered abnormal (hyperinsulinemia) with a peak $> 80 \, \mu U/ml$ associated with a $\Sigma > 200 \, \mu U/ml$. Controls were 29 normal weight subjects, aged 2.7–13.0 years. ANOVA, Student-Newman-Keuls' test, chi-square, or Fisher's exact test, coefficient of linear correlation were calculated.

Results

No differences were seen in blood glucose and IRI between patients and controls. In all patients and in subgroups B and C, Σ C-p was higher than in controls; both Σ IRI ($p = 0.006$) and Σ C-p ($p = 0.02$) (similar to controls, $p = 0.04$) were positively related to the age of patients and displayed greater levels in subgroup C with respect those of subgroup A (Table 1).

Σ IRI and Σ C-p levels were positively correlated both in patients and in controls ($p < 0.02$). In all patients as well as in subgroups B and C blood glucose levels were positively related to IRI levels ($p < 0.02$). The prevalence of GT impairment and hyperinsulinemia tends to increase with to the age of the patients (Table 2).

The individual mean of ferritin levels measured during the 3 years before the test was positively related to both Σ blood glucose and Σ IRI ($p = 0.01$) and negatively to the duration of pump application ($p < 0.02$).

Table 1. Peak (*P*) and sum of values during the OGTT (Σ) of circulating blood glucose, insulin, and C-peptide levels in polytransfused thalassemia major patients (evaluated as whole population and subdivided according to age) and in controls

| | Controls | All | Patients with thalassemia major | | |
			< 8 years	8–14 years	> 14 years
BG	P 144.2 ± 23.8 (29)	139.7 ± 26.5 (136)	141.4 ± 33.4 (14)	140.8 ± 21.6 (60)	138.1 ± 29.2 (62)
(mg/dl)	Σ 510.4 ± 65.4	537.7 ± 82.6	515.9 ± 90.0	540.4 ± 73.4	540.0 ± 89.7
IRI	P 45.1 ± 20.9 (29)	52.4 ± 32.5 (133)	39.5 ± 35.3 (14)	52.7 ± 28.2 (58)	55.2 ± 35.4 (61)
(µU/ml)	Σ 108.8 ± 48.3	124.7 ± 58.7	90.6 ± 49.4*	122.7 ± 59.9	134.4 ± 57.3*
C-p	P 4.02 ± 2.13 (15)	8.60 ± 7.39 (126)	5.54 ± 4.06 (13)	8.78 ± 6.00 (56)	9.11 ± 8.40 (57)
(nmol/l)	k 10.68 ± 5.51	23.34 ± 15.36 ##	13.17 ± 7.15 **	23.85 ± 16.3 #	25.16 ± 15.0 ## **

* p < 0.01; ** p < 0.02; # p < 0.05 and ## p < 0.01 vs controls. *BG*, Blood glucose; *IRI*, insulin; *C-p*, C-peptide.
Figures in brackets represent number of subjects.

Table 2. Number of controls and of polytransfused thalassemia major patients with an impairment of glucose tolerance and/or β-pancreatic function (for explanations see text)

| | Controls | Patients | | |
		< 8 years	8–14 years	> 14 years
a- One blood glucose level	6/29	2/11	10/42	9/39
b- Two blood glucose levels	0/29*	1/11	5/42	6/39*
c- Peak and Σ IRI values increased	1/29	1/11	4/42	6/39
a or b + c	0/29	0/11	5/42	5/39

* p = 0.029

Conclusion

The normal values of blood glucose, IRI and C-p levels during the OGTT, and the persistence of correlations between IRI and C-p levels, as well as between both IRI and C-p levels and chronological age, show that PF in the whole Th patient population was not impressively impaired. A reduced GT was sporadically observed; its prevalence was higher than in controls and increased with age. C-peptide is equimolecularly produced with insulin; its increased levels in Th patients older than 8 years with respect to controls, as well as the relationship between blood glucose and IRI levels, could reflect a slight insulin resistance, confirming previous data [8, 9]. A high ferritin level seems to be a risk factor for hyperinsulinemia and reduced GT.

References

1. Lassman MN, Genel M, Wise JK, Hendler R, Felig P (1974) Carbohydrate homeostasis and pancreatic islet cell function in thalassemia. Ann intem Med 80: 65–69
2. Costin G, Kogut MD, Hyman CB, Ortega JA (1977) Carbohydrate metabolism and pancreatic islet-cell function in thalassemia major. Diabetes 26: 230–240
3. Zuppinger K, Molinari B, Hirt A, Imbach P, Gugler E, Tonz O, Zurbrugg RP (1979) Increased risk of diabetes mellitus in beta-thalassemia major due to iron overload. Helv Pediatr Acta 34: 197–207
4. Capra L, Atti G, De Sanctis V, Candini G (1983) Glucose tolerance and chelation therapy in patients with thalassemia major. Haematologica (Pavia) 1: 63–67
5. Cavallo L, Acquafredda A, Bratta P, Schettini F (1985) Alterazioni della tolleranza glicidica e della funzione β-pancreatica in thalassemici major politrasfusi clinicamente prepuberi. Haematologica (Pavia) [Suppl] 1: 121–122
6. Livadas DP, Economou E, Sofroniadou K, Fotiadou-Pappa H, Van Melle GD, Temler E, Felber JP (1987) A study of beta-cell function after glucagon stimulation in thalassemia major treated by high transfusion program. Clin Endocrinol (Oxf) 27: 485–490
7. De Sanctis V, Zurlo MG, Senesi E, Boffa C, Cavallo L, Di Gregorio F (1988) Insulin-dependent diabetes mellitus in thalassemia. Arch Dis Child 63: 58–62
8. Merkel PA, Simonson DC, Amiel SA, Plewe G, Sherwin RS, Pearson HA, Tamborlane WV (1988) Insulin resistance and hyperinsulinemia in patients with thalassemia major treated by hypertransfusion. N Engl J Med 318: 809–814
9. Jones TW, Boulware SD, Caprio S, Merkel P, Amiel SA, Pearson HA, Aherwin RS, Tamborlane WV (1993) Correction of hyperinsulinemia by glyburide treatment in nondiabetic patients with thalassemia major. Pediatr Res 33: 497–500

β-Cell Glucose Non-sensing in Patients with Thalassemia major and Glucose Intolerance

G. Petrou, M. Makri, A. Armoni, B. E. Spiliotis, and T. K. Alexandrides

Diabetes mellitus (DM), a relatively frequent complication in patients with thalassemia major (β-thal), is usually attributed to insulin deficiency due to islet β-cell loss because of toxic effects of iron deposited in the pancreatic islets [1–4]. There is also evidence for insulin resistance in peripheral tissues that precedes the development of diabetes [5–8]. A prospective long-term study of ours (6 years) of 60 patients with β-thal (unpublished data) agrees with previous data in the literature [8] showing that insulin resistance becomes evident in the pubertal period and progressively increases with age. Since in type-I and type-II DM the earliest finding in the prediabetic state is the diminished first-phase response of insulin to glucose infusion (IVGTT), while the insulin response to i.v. arginine, i.v. glucagon, oral glucose tolerance (OGTT) and i.v. tolbutamide is preserved or slightly impaired, this has been interpreted as decreased β-cell glucose non-sensing [9]. The purpose of this study was to investigate the possibility that there is also β-cell glucose non-sensing in the prediabetic state in β-thal.

Materials and Methods

We studied four groups of patients as follows: group 1 consisted of ten β-thal patients with DM (mean age: 26.9 years); group 2 was 13 β-thal patients with impaired glucose tolerance (mean age: 22.6 years); group 3 was 14 β-thal patients with normal glucose tolerance (mean age: 16 years); group 4 was 17 normal controls (mean age 26 years).

The tests performed were a 3-h OGTT (1.75 g glucose/kg body wt.), intravenous glucagon (1 mg), and glucose infusion (0.5 g/kg body wt.). Glucose, insulin, and C-peptide levels were determined at the following time points before/after administration:
- OGTT: 0, 30, 60, 90, 120, and 180 min
- Glucagon: 0, 2, 4, 6, 8, and 20 min
- IVGTT: –15, 0, 2, 3, 5, 10, 10, and 30 min

S. Andò et al. (Eds.)
Endocrine Disorders in Thalassemia
© Springer-Verlag Berlin Heidelberg 1995

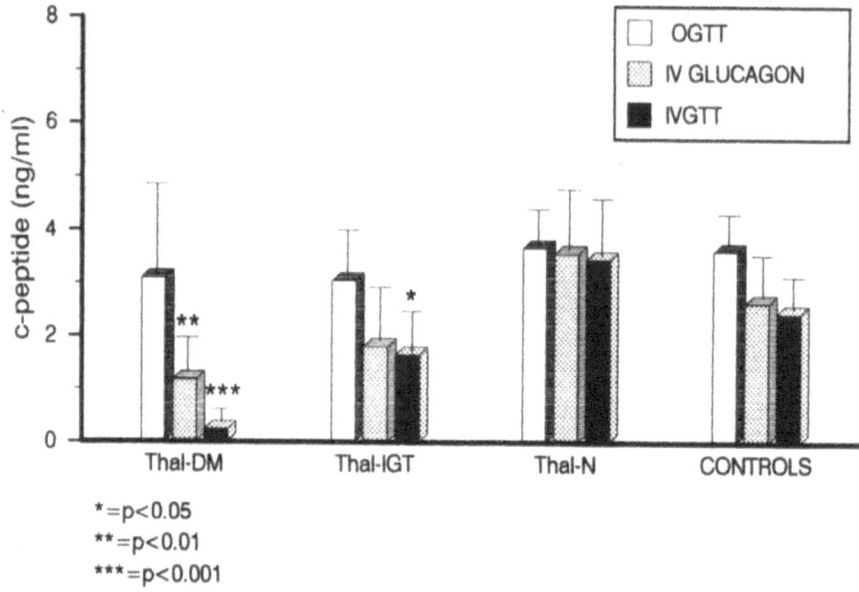

Fig. 1. C-peptide responses after OGTT, i. v. glucagon, and IVGTT in the four study groups.
Results for OGTT and i. v. glucagon are shown as the increase in the C-peptide levels over the basal
levels. The IVGTT results show the first-phase response over basal (i. e., the mean of the response
at 2, 3, and 5 min minus the mean of −15 and 0 min). The p values represent the significance of the
difference of the study groups as compared with normal controls

Biochemical Measurements

Plasma glucose was measured according to the glucose oxidase method, with a
glucose analyzer. Plasma concentration of insulin and C-peptide were measured by
double-antibody radioimmunoassay (Diagnostic Products).

Statistics

We performed two-tailed Student's unpaired t-tests for comparisons of two groups
and analysis of variance (ANOVA) for comparisons between three or more groups.

Results

Figure 1 shows the C-peptide response and Figure 2 the insulin response to the
three provocative tests (OGTT, glucagon, and IVGTT) in the four groups studied.
The C-peptide and insulin response after OGTT were similar in all four groups of
patients. In the i. v. glucagon test, the C-peptide and insulin response were significantly diminished only in the · β–thal DM patients as compared with normal

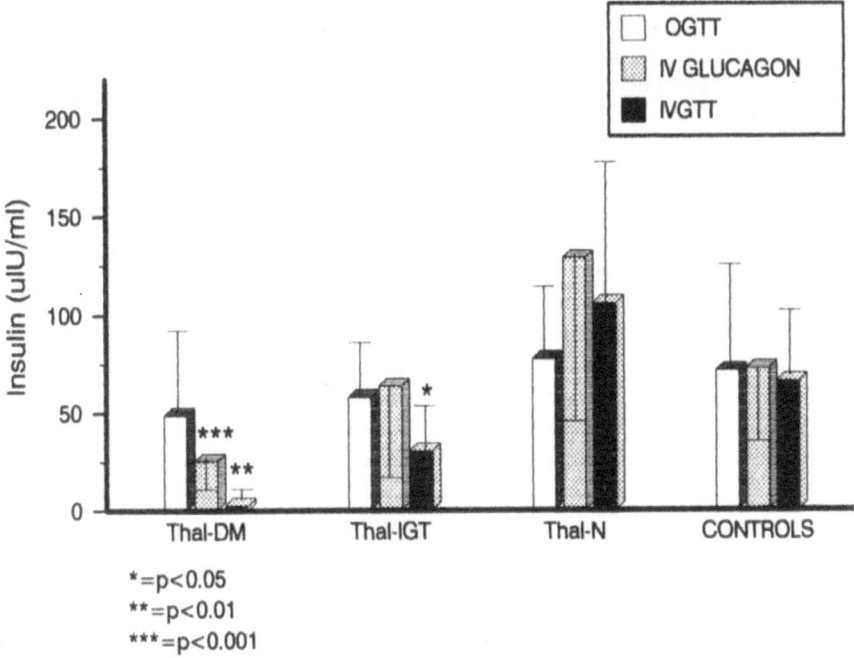

Fig. 2. Insulin responses after OGTT, i. v. glucagon, and IVGTT in the four study groups. Results for OGTT and i. v. glucagon are shown as the increase in the insulin levels over the basal levels. The IVGTT results show the first-phase response over basal (i. e., the mean of the response at 2, 3, and 5 min minus the mean of –15 and 0 min). The *p* values represent the significance of the difference of the study groups as compared with normal controls

controls. During the IVGTT the C-peptide and insulin responses were significantly diminished in the β-thal patients with impaired glucose tolerance and almost completely absent in the five β-thal patients who required no therapy for their mild DM. It became evident after i. v. glucagon stimulation in the ten β-thal DM patients that there is still a considerable C-peptide and insulin response, even though, in addition to the five patients with mild DM, this group also included five with severe DM.

Discussion

As is evident from our results, β-thal patients with impaired glucose tolerance do not have significantly decreased levels of insulin and C-peptide after OGTT or i. v. glucagon as compared with normal controls, but they do have a significant decrease in insulin and C-peptide levels after IVGTT. Of note is the observation that β-thal patients with mild DM have normal C-peptide and insulin responses after OGTT, while the same patients show almost a complete disappearance of the first-phase insulin response after IVGTT. It is also interesting that the five mild DM β-thal patients, together with an additional five β-thal patients with severe DM, showed a significant response in insulin and C-peptide secretion after i. v. glucagon.

Our data suggest that, similar to what occurs in type-I and type-II DM in patients without β-thal, there is a progressive loss of the first-phase response of insulin to i.v. glucose, and this first-phase response completely disappears with the onset of DM. This is analogous to what occurs in the prediabetic state in type-I [9] and type-II DM [10]. These data can be interpreted as showing that β-thal patients with DM have a significant number of β-cells that are able to respond to oral glucose with virtually normal insulin and C-peptide levels, while having lost the first-phase response of insulin to i. v. glucose, suggesting that the β-cell does not recognize hyperglycemia; i. e., it has a glucose-sensing dysfunction.

From these observations, we conclude that, as in the case of type-I and type-II DM, islet β-cells of patients with thalassemia major lose glucose sensing early in the process of the development of diabetes. In practical terms, this observation may be important for β-thal patients, in that the impairment of glucose sensing may be partially reversed, as has been shown in type-II DM when euglycemia was achieved [11].

References

1. Lassman MN, Genel M, Wise JK, Hendler R, Felig P (1974) Carbohydrate homeostasis and pancreatic islet cell function in thalassemia. Ann Intern Med 80: 65–69
2. McIntosh N (1976) Endocrinopathy in thalassemia major. Arch Dis child 51: 195–201
3. Saudek CD, Hemm RM, Peterson CM (1977) Abnormal glucose tolerance in β-thalassemia major. Metabolism 26: 43–52
4. Zuppinger K, Molinari B, Hirt A et al. (1979) Increased risk of diabetes mellitus in beta-thalassemia major due to iron overload. Helv Paediatr Acta 34: 197–207
5. Flynn DM, Fairney A, Jackson D, Clayton BE (1976) Hormonal changes in thalassemia major. Arch Dis Child 51: 828–836
6. Costin G, Kogut MD, Hyman C, Ortega JA (1977) Carbohydrate metabolism and pancreatic islet-cell function in thalassemia major. Diabetes 26: 230–240
7. Dandona P, Hussain MAM, Varghese Z, Politis D, Flynn DM, Hoffbrand AV (1983) Insulin resistance and iron overload. Ann Clin Biochem 20: 77–79
8. Merkel PA, Simonson DC, Amiel SA et al. (1988) Insulin resistance and hyperinsulinemia in patients with thalassemia major treated by hypertransfusion. N Engl J Med 318: 809–814
9. Ganda OP, Srikanta S, Brink SJ et al. (1984) Differential sensitivity to β-cell secretagogues in "early" type-I diabetes mellitus. Diabetes 33: 516–521
10. Brunzell JD, Robertson RP, Lerner RL et al. (1979) Relationship between fasting plasma glucose levels and insulin secretion during intravenous glucose tolerance tests. J Clin Endocrinol Metab 42: 222–229
11. Robertson RP (1989) Type-II diabetes, glucose "non-sense", and islet desensitization. Diabetes 38: 1501–1505

Secondary Diabetes mellitus in Thalassemic Patients

M. Karagiorga-Lagana, A. Chatziliami, A. Katsantoni,
F. Karabatsos, C. Fragodimitri, G. Tapaki, J. Jousef, M. Giannaki,
and A. Al-Qadreh

Introduction

Diabetes mellitus is a common complication in patients with thalassemia major (TM). The aim of this study was to evaluate the incidence of insulin-dependent diabetes mellitus (IDDM) and impaired glucose metabolism in patients with TM and to identify the effects of transfusional hemosiderosis, chronic liver damage, and positive family history on glucose metabolism. An approach to diabetic microangiopathy was made by detecting microalbuminuria, an early indicator of diabetic nephropathy, in the patients with IDDM and impaired glucose tolerance.

Patients and Methods

Three hundred ninety-two patients are being regularly followed in the Thalassemia Unit at The Aghia Sophia Children's Hospital in Athens. Nine patients (2,3%) have developed IDDM. A total of 231 thalassemics aged 13 years and above were studied for glucose tolerance by the oral glucose tolerance test (OGTT), performed and evaluated according to WHO criteria [12]. The patients were transfused to maintain the pretransfusion Hb between 9.5 and 10.5 g/dl and were chelated with desferrioxamine (DFO) subcutaneously. Serum ferritin, measured by the microparticle enzyme immunoassay technique (ABBOTT), was used as an indirect index for the degree of hemosiderosis. Liver function was evaluated according to alanine aminotransferase (SGP-T) values, measured by standard methods (normal range 5–45 U/l). All patients were screened for hepatitis B and C markers.

Microalbuminuria was estimated by nephelometry. A value of more than 30–140 mg/l of microalbumin in 3-h morning collections (after an overnight fast) was considered to represent microalbuminuria. All patients with IDDM and those with an impaired oral glucose tolerance test (IOGTT) were examined at least twice.

The coexistence of other endocrinopathies (uncompensated hypothyroidism, primary or secondary hypogonadism, hypoparathyroidism) was recorded and a family history of DM in first- and second-degree relatives was sought from the patients' clinical records. All data are presented as mean values ± standard deviation (SD). Statistical analysis was evaluated with the Student's t-test.

S. Andò et al. (Eds.)
Endocrine Disorders in Thalassemia
© Springer-Verlag Berlin Heidelberg 1995

Results

Insulin-dependent diabetes mellitus has developed in nine of the 392 patients (2.3%) (group I). Forty-one of the 231 patients (17%) had an IOGTT (group II). The OGTT was normal in 190 of the 231 thalassemics (83%). Of these, 65 patients matched for age and sex with patients of group II were used as controls (group III). The mean age of the patients in groups I, II, and III was 21.6 ± 2.4, 21 ± 4.3, and 20.3 ± 3.1 years, respectively, and was comparable. The mean age at the onset of IDDM was 16 ± 3 years. The duration of IDDM ranges from 4 to 12 years. The mean age at the onset of IOGTT was 18 ± 4 years.

Mean serum ferritin levels, age at start of iron chelation with SCDFO, the number of patients splenectomized, and the mean age at splenectomy in groups I, II, and III are presented in Table 1. The difference in ferritin levels between group I and II was significant at the $p = 0.03$ level but not between group II and the controls (group III). The patients with IDDM had started iron chelation with DFO at a later age than those with IOGTT or the controls. This difference was statistically significant ($p = 0.03$).

The mean SGP-T values and the percentage of patients infected with hepatitis B (HBV) and C virus (HCV) in the three groups are presented in Table 2. The difference in SGP-T between groups I and II was significant at the 0.02 level and

Table 1. Serum ferritin, age at start of DFO, and age at splenectomy in groups I, II, and III of thalassemic patients ($n = 9$, 41 and 65 respectively)

	Group I	p	Group II	p	Group III
Ferritin (ng/ml)	6022 ± 775	0.03	4200 ± 2830	NS	3790 ± 2121
Age at start of DFO (years)	12.1 ± 2	0.03	10.8 ± 3	NS	10 ± 3
Splenectomy (n)	5		12		21
Age at splenectomy (years)	13.7 ± 9	NS	12.7 ± 5	0.04	16 ± 4.5

DFO, Desferrioxamine, *NS*, nonsignificant

Table 2. SGP-T values and incidence of post-transfusion hepatitis B and C in the three groups of patients

	Group I	p	Group II	p	Group III
SGP-T (U/l)	192 ± 148	0.02	107 ± 97	0.01	72 ± 55
Heapatitits B					
(n)	9/9		35/41		58/65
(%)	100		85		89
Hepatitits C					
(n)	8/9		22/41		24/65
(%)	89		54		37

Table 3. Incidence of endocrinopathies in the three groups of patients

Group	I $n = 9$	II $n = 41$	III $n = 65$
Hypothyroidism	4	12	9
Hypoparathyroidism	2	3	4
Hypogonadism	6	22	27
No encrinopathy	1 (11%)	13 (31%)	36 (54%)

between group II and the controls (group III) as well at the 0.01 level. A high percentage of our patients were infected with HBV and HCV. Microalbuminuria was detected in only one male patient with IDDM 12 years after onset. None of the patients with IOGTT (group II) had microalbuminuria.

Hypogonadism (primary or secondary), hypothyroidism, and hypoparathyroidism are usual complications in TM. The coexistence of more than one endocrinopathy in the same patient is not a rare phenomenon (Table 3). The most frequent one is hypogonadism.

A family history of DM type II was present in 44, 29, and 26% of the patients in groups I and II and the controls (group III), respectively.

Discussion

Diabetes mellitus is a frequent complication in patients with thalassemia major. The prevalence of IDDM in our thalassemics is 2.3% (nine of 392 patients). This is in agreement with the literature [2, 4, 6, 11], although percentages up to 22% have been reported [1, 13, 14]. The incidence of impaired glucose tolerance was lower (17%) in our patients than in other studies [2, 10, 13, 14]. The mean age at the onset of IDDM was 16 ± 3 years, as in most other studies [2, 4, 6, 13].

The pathogenesis of diabetes mellitus complicating thalassemia major has not yet been completely elucidated. Iron overload plays an important role by damaging the pancreatic β-cell, with consequent insulin deficiency, and the liver cell, with consequent insulin resistance [2, 4, 7, 8, 10, 11, 14]. In this study patients with IDDM had a heavier iron load, as indicated by their higher serum ferritin levels, and had started iron chelation with desferrioxamine later than those with impaired or normal OGTT.

Chronic hepatitis and cirrhosis is another critical factor for the development of glucose intolerance and, in time, isulin-dependent diabetes [1, 3, 5]. Costin et al. [3] suggested that insulin resistance and hyperglucagonemia secondary to cirrhosis, rather than insulinopenia, are the main factors which lead to diabetes during the course of thalassemia major. Liver damage caused by iron toxicity and viral infections (hepatitis B and, mainly, C) was more prominent in our thalassemics with IDDM and IOGTT than in controls.

In our study, a family history of diabetes was present in 44% of patients with insulin-dependent diabetes and in 29% with IOGTT. Saudek et al. [10] found that

75 % of their thalassemics with a positive family history for diabetes had abnormal glucose tolerance. The importance of genetic predisposition has been confirmed also by others [2, 4].

Nephropathy is the major complication of IDDM, developing in approximately 35 % of all type-1 diabetic patients. The incidence of this complication is nil in the first 5 years of IDDM and peaks in the second decade of the disease [9]. Micro-albuminuria is strongly predictive of late nephropathy [3], so it may be considered a suitable marker for early detection of renal dysfunction. Microalbuminuria was observed in only one patients with IDDM after 12 years on insulin treatment.

The coexistence of diabetes mellitus or impaired glucose tolerance with other endocrinopathies in the same thalassemic patient has been described also by other authors [4, 10,11].

The results of this study show that iron overload, which damages to a varying extent the pancreatic and liver cells, liver damage caused by viral infections, and a family history of diabetes mellitus are very important risk factors for the develop-ment of impaired glucose metabolism. It is hoped that the majority of thalassemic patients will be protected from developing diabetes by early and regular iron chelation, routine vaccination with the hepatitis-B vaccine, and screening of blood donors for hepatitits B and C. The OGTT should be performed yearly, at least after the age of 12 years, or even earlier in all cases with a family history of DM, for timely identification of those with IOGTT, in order to provide them with the appro-priate intervention concerning diet, exercise, and probably oral antidiabetics.

References

1. Atti G, Capra L, De Sanctis V, Vullo C, Bagni B (1983) Beta-cell function assessed by plasma C-peptide evaluation in diabetic thalassemic patients. Helv Paediatr Acta 38: 123–132
2. Capra L, Atti G, De Sanctis V, Candini G (1983) Glucose tolerance and chelation therapy in patients with thalassemia major. Haematologica (Pavia) 68: 63–67
3. Costin G, Kogut M, Hyman C, Ortega J (1977) Carbohydrate metabolism and pancreatic islet-cell function in thalassaemia major. Diabetes 26: 230–240
4. De Sanctis V, Zurlo M, Senesis E, Boffa C, Cavallo L, Di Gregorio F (1988) Insulin-dependent diabetes in thalassaemia. Arch Dis Child 63: 58–62
5. De Sanctis V, D'Ascola G, Wonke B (1987) Long-term follow-up study on the development of diabetes mellitus in optimally treated β-thalassemia patients. In: Sirchia G, Zanella A (eds) Thalassemia today. The Mediterranean experience. Centro Transfusionale Ospedale Maggiore Policlinico di Milano, Milan, pp 289–292
6. Kattamis C, Ladis V, Jacovides N, Theodoridis C (1989) Glucose tolerance and insulin response in patients with thalassemia (Abstr 375) Eur J Clin Invest 19: A67
7. Lassman M, O'Brien R, Plarson A, Wise J, Donebedian R, Felig B, Gene L (1974) Endocrine evaluation in thalassemia major. Ann NY Acad Sci 232: 226–237
8. Merkel P, Simonson D, Amiels S, Plewe G, Sherwin R, Pearson H, Tamborlane W (1988) Insulin resistance and hyperinsulinemia in patients with thalassemia major treated by hypertransfusion. N Engl J Med 318: 809–814
9. Mogensen CE (1987) Microalbuminuria as a predictor or clinical diabetic nephropathy, Kidney Int 31: 673–679
10. Saudek C, Hemm C, Peterson C (1977) Abnormal glucose tolerance in β-thalassemia major. Metabolism 26: 43–52

11. Vullo C, De Sanctis V, Katz M, Wonke B, Hoffbrandt A, Bagni B, Torresani T, Tolis G, Masiero M, Di Palma A, Borgatti L (1990) Endocrine abnormalities in thalassemia. Ann NY Acad Sci 612: 293–310
12. WHO (1980) Impaired glucose tolerance and diabetes – WHO criteria. Br Med J 281: 1512–1513
13. Wonke B, De Sanctis V (1992) Glucose intolerance and diabetes in multiply transfused patients with thalassaemia major. International Mediterranean Conference on Endocrine Disorders in Thalassemia, Consenza, p 25
14. Zuppinger K, Molinari B, Hirt A, Imbach P, Gugler E, Tonz O, Zurbrugg R (1979) Increased risk of diabetes mellitus in beta- thalassemia major due to iron overload. Helv paediatr Acta 34: 197–207

Subject Index

Springer-Verlag
and the Environment

We at Springer-Verlag firmly believe that an international science publisher has a special obligation to the environment, and our corporate policies consistently reflect this conviction.

We also expect our business partners – paper mills, printers, packaging manufacturers, etc. – to commit themselves to using environmentally friendly materials and production processes.

The paper in this book is made from low- or no-chlorine pulp and is acid free, in conformance with international standards for paper permanency.